FIRST PRINCIPLES

Oral Airway Functional Maldevelopment Syndrome (OAFMS)

The Health Continuum

SCOTT WUSTENBERG

How a Small Problem in Early Life Creates Havoc Across Time

The link between Sleep, Breathing and the Airway that Drive Human development to health or disease.

Disclaimer

First Principles aims to make the connections and links of already existing research available in one place to the medical and scientific community. This book is purely for the educational purpose of creating greater awareness and discussion within the medical community. This book does not cater to the needs of individual patients and is designed to support, not replace, the relationship that exists between a patient/site visitor and his/her existing physician. This book is not a therapy book, nor does it contain any treatment options or suggestions, it is a unique collection of standing medical research.

Copyright © 2023 by Dr. Scott Wustenberg

Trademarks® 2023 OSAH - Optimal Sleep Airway Health, The Infinite Health Continuum, by Dr Scott Wustenberg

All rights reserved. No part of this book may be reproduced or used in any manner without written permission of the copyright owner except for the use of quotations in a book review. For more information, please address: maria@notredpen.com.au

First published in 2023

Wustenberg, Dr. Scott

Cover design: Natasha Williams - DAZED Designs dazed-designs.com

Editing: Maria Smith - Not the Red Pen

Formatting: Natasha Williams - DAZED Designs dazed-designs.com

Prologue

I would like to take you on a journey, a thought experiment if you will. We will take it together and expand our understanding of human health and development from just after conception through until later in life where we see symptoms develop. The purpose of this book to help the lay person and the practitioner alike see that life is a continuum, that issues that are picked up on in later life are there because they were missed early and have morphed into something that today's health practitioners see through the lens of their specialty and not as part of a greater issue in the making. I hope that I can convince the medical fraternities to become more collaborative especially in a child's earlier life, since the purpose of earlier intervention is to save human suffering and improve our society as a whole.

I will discuss the importance of sleep, its interaction with health in general, craniofacial development and its impact on function and form of the human, the impact of epigenetics during pregnancy on the neurological as well as facial development of the child, how primitive reflexes drive development of the infant towards adulthood and what it would look like if the primitive reflexes do not integrate efficiently. We will look at how this will increase the likely outcome of different diagnoses such as ADHD, snoring and sleep apnoea, hypertension, and cardiovascular disease, while diabetes and stroke is also highly associated with this journey.

Without a hint of cynicism, we can accept that from a purely financial point of view maintaining the status quo is of benefit for the different practitioners that see the patient across the course of their symptom development, however this is not the best or most efficient use of resources, nor does it help the human be their best self. In fact, this separation of healthcare into modules that the human interfaces with as symptoms patterns develop at different ages of life is accepted as normal and is often put down to as human ageing. This is not the case and enhances the amount of human suffering and may very well decrease the quality of life experienced or decrease the quantity of this life as well.

Think therefore, from a financial perspective that if my thesis is correct and we intervene early and often to re-establish normal developmental trajectory for the infant, how much money can be redeployed in more meaningful directions, how much suffering can be averted, how many man hours of productive capacity can be saved. Oral Craniofacial maldevelopment walks hand in hand with non-neurotypical outcomes as we will see including Anxiety, OCD, depression, ADHD as well as dementia as an endpoint. Saving the suffering early and preventing inflammatory upregulation has to be a goal of any human flourishing focused, health practitioner, let alone the goal of every parent.

Human flourishing is determined by the development of the brain. The purpose of the brain is a bit of an underwhelming surprise. It is to maintain survival of the organism in the immediacy, as against more exceptional functions attributed to our species. What I mean is: the brain cares about dealing with threat now, this second, not the threat that may occur next week or further to the future. If there is a tiger in front of me, I am not worried about the dangers of diabetes that could kill me in 10 years' time, as the tiger can kill me now. Thus, we must view unconscious behaviours, reflexes, and decisions of the brain from this viewpoint, as sometimes immediate survival may be at odds and be contradictory to long term survival actions.

Because the brain is a pattern recognising machine, we consume data and try to find meaning to everything including our "purpose". When you strip all the hyperbole away, survival is at the root of all flourishing. Therefore, all of our systems, be it genetic, neurocognitive, higher behaviour functions such as love, digestion, detoxification and so many more are influenced or directed by this goal (immediate survival) or "purpose".

Ultimately true survival is expressed by getting your genes into the next generation and raising the offspring in safety to their maturity so that this act can be repeated. Along the way survival is demonstrated by making conscious and/or unconscious decisions that lead to actions that maintain the organism in its immediacy. Prepartum or in the infantile post-partum state then this survival is demonstrated by hardwired reflexogenic action that has been programmed from previous specious success to cause the adult to look after it. Unconscious decisions/actions do not consider the future, only the threat/stimuli in front of it now.

Because the Human is multi-layered, complicated, and never the same neurocognitively we have deduced generalised rules that must always be sacrosanct to understand ourselves, principles that must be applied by the human (mostly unconsciously as they are not aware of these rules) to bend energy, in time and space to bring consciousness into being and produce survival. These rules help us function at an optimum level and will be explained below.

There are **4 Rules** with which I view all patients I see, their symptoms, patterns, and behaviours. If I'm honest, Rule 3 and 4 are subsets of Rule 2 but they are so important I emphasise them so that the person I'm explaining them to starts altering how they view themselves, their symptoms and their actions to improve themselves.

1

The Rules of Being Human

Rule 1

Everything occurring in the human is done so by the brain/central nervous system - All symptoms, all actions, and sensations you can observe (excluding immediate trauma) are done to you on purpose by the brain as the alternate (such as death) is worse, when viewed from the "purpose of the brain" viewpoint, that being survival.

At least this is how it initially starts. There is a slight exception to this rule that can occur in the long term due to Neuroplasticity. Plasticity starts from the survival point of view, and can create issues that perpetuate loops of negativity, driving development away from optimal.

Rule 2

Everything is in some way shape or form a resource management issue. If you don't have enough resources, if they are poorly distributed, or even too much of a resource (Perhaps leading to toxicity) then outcomes will be suboptimal, and compensation will occur to maintain survival of the organism.

Think too much iron- this can cause oxidative stress and liver damage, or if you consume too little water then the brain loses capacity to think clearly, hallucination and deliriousness can occur with a worst case of death in the extreme scenario.

Rule 3

Everything occurring in the body and especially the brain is affected by sleep, both the quality and quantity- if you don't sleep you don't heal. In fact, if you don't sleep you will die[i].

While sleep is arguably a subset of 2. above it is so important it needs to be noted as a specific rule.

Although the absolute biological function of sleep remains uncertain, the consequences of sleep deprivation are well-described and are reported to be detrimental to cognitive function and affective well-being. Sleep is imperative for all systems to function, including but not limited to growth, repair, and detoxification[ii].

Rule 4

Everything occurring in the body and the brain is affected by Breathing - if you don't breathe well you don't heal. If you don't breathe for long enough you get brain damage and can die, the airway must be defended.

Again, we can all appreciate that gas exchange is a subset of Rule 2 above, but it is so important to life that it has its own rule. Breathing itself is more than just the act of oxygen and carbon dioxide exchange, at a minimum it is one of the few tools the human can use consciously to affect the vagus nerve and calm our nervous system or if distressed ramp up the CNS for survival. It is also essential for metabolism to occur, for energy production and burning in the mitochondria via respiration.

The rules are constant and occur in all of us and apply at every second of our life. There are further principles that determine how we function and behave, the output of the brain so to speak which we will pepper through as we go, but it is essential to understand the four rules above when considering why a compensation occurs or a behaviour or a symptom is apparent.

Survival is the most important thing the brain must do moment by moment and it gives a rationale on how to apply Jaak Panksepp's work Affective neuroscience. Jaak details the primary emotions, Seeking, Lust, Fear, Rage, Panic, hunger, and play which underpin our survival behaviours and lead to more complex secondary and tertiary emotions and behavioural outputs. If there is no rational way to survive then there is no point to seeking food when one is hungry. Similarly, to truly survive your genes must get into the next generation, therefore you must seek sex which is driven by lust. The tertiary level emotion is Love; it is not essential for survival but it makes relationships better.

The primary emotions allow the human to survive, but further they allow us the basis of complex emotion to interface with the world and other people.

Before we get to the meat of my thesis, I think it important that the lay reader has some definitions and understanding of basic physiology so we can all be on the same page regardless of where you come from, for the clinician please feel free to skip these boring bits as you should already know this.

2

Respiration Basics

Breathing is the process of inhaling oxygen and exhaling carbon dioxide. It is essential for life because it allows the body to exchange gases with the environment and maintain proper levels of oxygen and carbon dioxide in the body.

Oxygen is essential for life because it is necessary for the body's cells to produce energy. When oxygen is inhaled into the body, it is taken up by the red blood cells and transported to the body's cells, where it is used in the process of cellular respiration. During cellular respiration, oxygen reacts with glucose (a simple sugar) to produce energy in the form of ATP (adenosine triphosphate). ATP is the primary source of energy for the body's cells and is used to fuel all the body's functions. Without oxygen, the body's cells cannot produce energy and will begin to die. Therefore, it is essential for the body to get a constant supply of oxygen from the environment.

Oxygen is also important for maintaining the body's pH balance and for supporting the immune system. It helps to neutralise harmful substances in the body, such as free radicals, which can cause damage to cells and lead to the development of diseases such as cancer. Oxygen also plays a vital role in the body's detoxification processes, helping to eliminate waste products and toxins from the body.

Although carbon dioxide is not essential for life in the same way that oxygen is, it plays an important role in the body's processes.

AEROBIC RESPIRATION

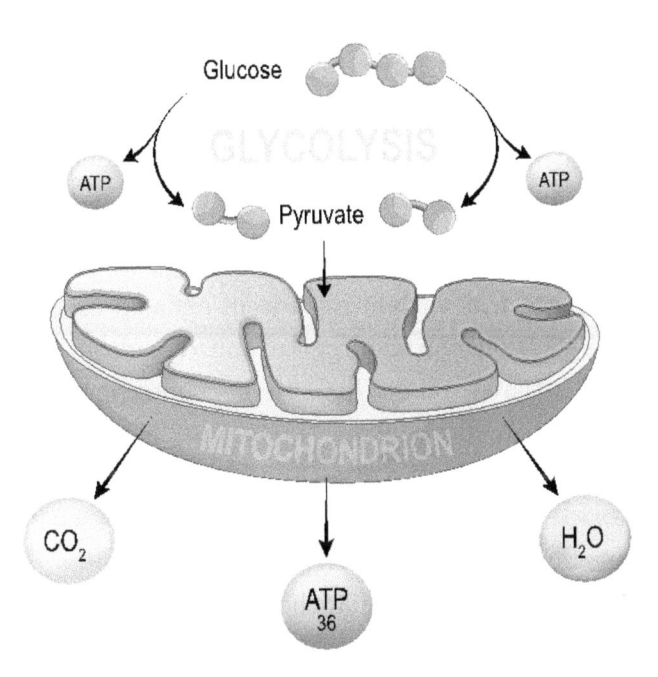

Diagram of Aerobic Respiration

Carbon dioxide is produced as a by-product of cellular respiration, the process by which the body's cells produce energy. During cellular respiration, oxygen reacts with glucose (a simple sugar) to produce energy in the form of ATP (adenosine triphosphate) and carbon dioxide as a waste product.

Carbon dioxide is a gas that is released into the bloodstream and transported to the lungs, where it is exhaled out of the body. The level of carbon dioxide in the body is carefully regulated by the respiratory system. Carbon dioxide has several important functions in the body. It helps to regulate the pH of the blood, ensuring that it stays at a neutral level. It also plays a role in the regulation of blood pressure and in the contraction and relaxation of smooth muscle tissue, such as in the walls of blood vessels.

The composition of the air we breathe is approximately 21% oxygen and 0.04% carbon dioxide. These proportions are essential for life, as oxygen is necessary for the body's cells to produce energy, while carbon dioxide is considered a waste product of cellular metabolism that must be eliminated from the body it is quite essential for human biology to function.

The concentration of carbon dioxide in exhaled air is typically higher than the concentration of carbon dioxide in the air we inhale. The normal range for the concentration of carbon dioxide in exhaled air is about 35-45 mm Hg (millimetres of mercury). This corresponds to a concentration of about 4.5-6% carbon dioxide. This is considerably more than the 0.04% intake and occurs due to the essential activity of respiratory chains working efficiently in our mitochondria, this is the basis of "metabolism".

The concentration of oxygen in the air is relatively constant, but the concentration of carbon dioxide can vary depending on several factors, including the level of pollution and the presence of plants, which absorb carbon dioxide and release oxygen during photosynthesis.

It is important to maintain a balance of carbon dioxide in the body. If the concentration of carbon dioxide in the blood becomes too high or too low, it can have negative effects on health. For example, if the concentration of carbon dioxide in the blood becomes too high, it can lead to a condition called acidosis, which can cause symptoms such as difficulty breathing, fatigue, and confusion. On the other hand, if the concentration of carbon dioxide in the blood becomes too low, it can lead to a condition called alkalosis, which can cause symptoms such as muscle twitching, tingling sensations, and confusion. Neither is good for the brain.

In summary, while oxygen is essential to produce energy and in the maintenance of life, carbon dioxide is an important by-product of energy production that plays a number of important roles in the body and without which respiration flounders. As an interesting thought point, carbon dioxide may very well be the end product by which the human actually burns fat out of the body and releases it when trying to lose weight. This indicates humans currently are the ultimate carbon capture systems as the western world gets fatter, and we should be encouraging carbon dioxide release for our own personal health.

3

The Bohr Effect

The Bohr effect refers to the effect of carbon dioxide and pH on the oxygen-binding capacity of haemoglobin, the protein in red blood cells that binds and transports oxygen in the body.

The Bohr effect was first described by Danish physiologist Christian Bohr in 1904. He observed that when the concentration of carbon dioxide in the blood increases, the affinity of haemoglobin for oxygen decreases. This means that haemoglobin is less able to bind and transport oxygen to the body's tissues. The Bohr effect is caused by the pH of the blood. Carbon dioxide is built up as part of cellular metabolism that is produced when the body's cells use oxygen to produce energy. As the concentration of carbon dioxide in the blood increases, the pH of the blood becomes more acidic, which causes the affinity of haemoglobin for oxygen to decrease. The Bohr effect is important because it allows the body to adjust the oxygen-binding capacity of haemoglobin in response to changes in the level of carbon dioxide in the blood. This helps to ensure that the body gets an adequate supply of oxygen to meet its energy needs, while also allowing it to get rid of excess carbon dioxide.

The Bohr effect is also involved in the regulation of blood pressure. When the blood vessels constrict, the level of carbon dioxide in the blood increases, which causes the affinity of haemoglobin for oxygen to decrease. This leads to an increase in the release of oxygen from haemoglobin, which helps to maintain blood pressure.

Breathing is controlled by the respiratory system, which includes the lungs, trachea, bronchi, and alveoli. When we breathe in, the muscles of the chest and diaphragm contract, causing the lungs to expand and draw in air. The air then travels through the trachea, bronchi, and alveoli, which are small air sacs in the lungs where gas exchange occurs. Oxygen from the air passes into the blood through the alveoli and is carried to the body's cells by the circulatory system. Carbon dioxide, a waste product of cellular metabolism, is exhaled out of the body. Breathing is important for maintaining a healthy body and mind. Proper breathing can help improve oxygen delivery to the body's cells, which can improve energy levels, brain function, and overall health. It can also help reduce stress and anxiety and promote relaxation. There are many different breathing techniques that can be used to promote relaxation and improve health, including deep breathing, diaphragmatic breathing, and belly breathing.

Sleep Basics

My idea is that the purpose of sleep (apart from the known basics) as humans do it, is to act as a heat sink for the brain. Kind of like a fan inside a computer server. The other purposes we know of include: organising the brain's learning capacity, stabilising emotions, growth and repair, detoxification as well as keeping memory organised so that the human can be in the present, understand the past and imagine a future.

Sleep is organised in 3 parts, Awake, then **NREM** (Non Rapid Eye Movement) which includes the below 4 stages as well as REM (Rapid Eye Movement).

There are four stages of NREM sleep

- **Stage 1**: This is the lightest stage of sleep, and it is easy to wake someone up during this stage. It is the transition between being awake and asleep, and it lasts for about 5-10 minutes.

- **Stage 2**: This is a deeper stage of sleep, and it is more difficult to wake someone up during this stage. It is the stage in which the body starts to relax and slow down. This stage lasts for about 20-25 minutes.
- **Stage 3**: This is the deepest and most restorative stage of sleep. It is the stage in which the body repairs and regenerates tissues, builds bone and muscle, and strengthens the immune system. This stage is also known as slow-wave sleep or delta sleep. It typically lasts for about 30-45 minutes.
- **Stage 4**: This is the final stage of sleep, and it is the most difficult to wake someone up from. It is similar to stage 3 in that it is a deep and restorative stage of sleep. It typically lasts for about 20-30 minutes.

Rapid Eye Movement (REM)

Rapid Eye Movement (REM) sleep is a stage of sleep that occurs after stage 4 sleep and is actually closer to Stage 1 and waking than it is too deep sleep, you must transition through Stage 2 and 1 to move to REM. It is characterised by the characteristic rapid eye movements, along with increased brain activity, and increased blood flow to the brain. During REM sleep, the brain is more active than during non-REM sleep and produces brain waves that are similar to those produced when a person is awake.

During REM sleep, the body becomes paralysed, and the person is unable to move. This is thought to be a protective mechanism that prevents the person from acting out their dreams. The paralysis can become dysregulated in some people and become over strong leading to airway collapse, snoring hypopneas, and apnoea, and all the many associated diseases that they cause. These are associated issues that start in utero which we will discuss later in the book. REM sleep is also known for its role in memory consolidation and the regulation of mood.

The first REM period typically occurs about 80-90 minutes after falling asleep and lasts for about 10 minutes. As the night progresses, the duration of REM sleep increases and the periods of non-REM sleep decreases. By the end of the night, a person may be in REM sleep for up to an hour.

The brain's activity changes during the different stages of sleep and can be measured using an electroencephalograph (EEG), which records the brain's electrical activity.

During stage 1 sleep, the brain waves are slower and less synchronised than when the person is awake. The brain produces alpha and theta waves, which are slower frequency waves. Alpha waves have a frequency of 8 to 12 Hz, while the Theta waves have a frequency of 4 to 8 Hz.

During stage 2 sleep, the brain waves become even slower and more synchronised. The brain produces sleep spindles, which are bursts of rapid brain activity, and K-complexes, which are sharp, single waves.

During stage 3 sleep, the brain produces slow, large delta waves. Delta waves have a frequency of 0.1 to 4 Hz

During stage 4 sleep, the brain continues to produce delta waves, which are even slower and larger than in stage 3 sleep. Delta waves have a frequency of 0.1 to 4 Hz

These are approximate ranges, and the exact frequencies can vary somewhat depending on the individual and the specific activity they are engaged in. It's also worth noting that these are just general ranges, and there can be some overlap between them. For example, a person may produce waves that fall into both the Theta and Alpha range.

It is important to note that the brain does not progress through the stages of sleep in a linear fashion. It will often go back and forth between the different stage's multiple times throughout the night.

Ageing and sleep

As people age, they tend to experience changes in their sleep patterns and sleep quality. These changes can include:

- Decreased total sleep time: Older adults tend to sleep less overall, and they may have difficulty falling asleep or staying asleep through the night.
- Changes in sleep stages: Older adults tend to spend less time in deep sleep (also known as slow-wave sleep) and more time in light sleep. This can lead to feelings of not being well-rested and can increase the risk of daytime sleepiness.
- Increased sleep disruption: Older adults may be more susceptible to sleep disruptions such as sleep apnoea, restless leg syndrome, and periodic limb movement disorder, which can further impair sleep quality.
- Changes in sleep-wake cycle: As people age, they may experience changes in their body's internal clock, which can affect their sleep-wake cycle and make it more difficult to fall asleep and wake up at the desired times.

Overall, ageing is associated with a number of changes in sleep patterns and sleep quality, and these changes can have a significant impact on an individual's health and well-being.

Obstructive sleep apnoea (OSA)

Obstructive sleep apnoea (OSA) is a sleep disorder that occurs when a person's airway becomes blocked during sleep, disrupting their breathing and preventing them from getting enough oxygen. OSA can affect all stages of sleep, but it is most likely to occur during stages 3 and 4, which are the deepest stages of sleep. During these stages, the muscles of the throat relax, and the airway can become narrow or collapse, causing the person to stop breathing for brief periods of time. This can cause the person to wake up frequently throughout the night, often without realising it, and can result in poor sleep quality and daytime sleepiness. OSA is a serious condition that can have serious health consequences if left untreated. We will discuss OSA in greater depth as we continue through this thesis.

It is important to get enough sleep and to have a regular sleep schedule in order to maintain good health. Getting insufficient sleep can have negative effects on physical and mental health, including an increased risk of developing conditions such as diabetes, heart disease, and obesity. It can also affect cognitive function, mood, and overall quality of life.

Sleep and Breathing

Sleep and Breathing are two major pillars to human health, both are resources that are essential in how the brain mange's your day-to-day stress versus thrive response. The golden rule is if you don't sleep, you don't heal, and everything in healing and health is affected by the quality of how you breath and the oxygen available to the brain, if there is a decrease in oxygenated blood supplied to the CNS, we see an increase in partially reduced oxygen species (**PROS**) production from the mitochondria which is demonstrated to contribute to neuronal damage during reoxygenation [iii].

Hopefully it is obvious that the developing infant brain is more vulnerable than the adult brain to reactive oxygen and reactive nitrogen species–mediated damage. Firstly, it is less stable and has a significantly higher metabolic demand as well as cellular turnover compared to the adult, it has high concentrations of unsaturated fatty acids, high rate of oxygen consumption, low concentrations of antioxidants, high content of metals catalysing free radical formation, and large proportion of sensitive immature cells[iv], all making for disaster if hypoxia occurs either acutely or repeatedly.

Oxidative stress is noted in the pathogenesis of neuronal cell death after exposure of the infant brain to hyperoxia, hypoxia/ischemia from sleep breathing issues as well as exposure to teratological agents and/or toxins, or from mechanical trauma as you might find in an intervention birthing process such as a forceps delivery. As it turns out the timing of our greatest vulnerability to **TBI** (traumatic brain injury) coincides with the peak of the brain growth spurts, including ischaemic injury.

I raise this as a significant concern as there are limited neuroprotective treatment strategies to combat oxidative stress in the clinical setting especially in infants let alone the foetus in the womb. The overweight adult with snoring (think hypopnea) or apnoea commonly doesn't even recognise they're in danger from oxidative damage, meaning that maintaining oxygen exchange capacity and a patent airway in the infant as well as in the adult is the most important strategy we have to thrive.

The Tongue

The tongue and its posture in the mouth and pharynx are an undervalued and often overlooked part of the oral apparatus that is essential for human survival. It plays an important role in swallowing, it affects dentofacial growth patterns, and craniofacial structural development[v] as well as in breathing capacity especially at night when the human is asleep. Tongue induced breathing faults are noted in deep sleep but especially in the rapid eye movement (REM) phase of sleep, when most sudden infant death occurs[vi], and more recently SADS, sudden adult death syndrome. SADS is highly controversial as it has before 2022 never been described as a disease syndrome and has been linked to COVID 19, Chronic Long Haul covid 19 complications or effects of the vaccination in a minority of people. While cause has not been established this disturbing event surely needs more investigation for mechanism, cause, and a treatment intervention to protect at risk individuals.

Tongue function, oral fascia, cranial structure, and their roles in health are topics that directly impacts on the capacity of breathing and oxygenation but passes very little scrutiny or investigation by readers of the medical literature. They can impact sleep quality and lead to stress responses in the infant that include cortisol and adrenaline release by the nervous system to maintain airway patency, as well as upregulation of the immune system and chemokine release. These have far reached impacts of human wellbeing both as infants, as well as through life as we will see.

Later we will discuss ankyloglossia, more commonly called tongue tie and try to bring attention to its impact, how poorly it is diagnosed and how little concern for its impact on human development is shown for dysfunction of the oral apparatus.

In the case of newborn infants and tongue tie, unless the tie is so severe and obvious causing the newborn much distress and a failure to thrive, then it seems almost that their problem is catalogued by whether the infant can bottle feed and if so, and they are putting on some weight then there is no problem and the oral restriction and its impact (or causative) neurological correlates are glossed over, their long term consequences including health disease growth (think speech dysfunction, orthodontics, ADHD anxiety hypertension, heart disease, diabetes or stroke) is completely ignored.

This is far from the truth, which we shall expand upon. Further, tongue tie in the older population is ignored as if it doesn't exist. But think, if it was missed in the child, then it continues as they grow to adulthood. It will metamorphosize into new and varied symptoms, in the adult not obviously associated with the tongue or mouth including neck and back Pain, postural irregularity amongst many others in the continuum of human life.

The Tongue as a problem is ignored

It's as if it's considered a problem only in children, and its connection to many other conditions is not making the literature. The literature is tries to make clear that tongue tie stops at about three or four years of age from a publication point, after breast feeding age is passed, papers about largely stop As it should be obvious to all, oral facial restriction, open bites, craniofacial maldevelopment, mouth breathing, snoring, and all the other symptoms of dysfunction still exist in the child regardless of attention paid by researchers and realistically are just getting entrenched in the nervous system, leading to a lifetime of growing ill health and diseases, many of which you might not consider to be linked to their beginning point in utero, or in the period not long after birth.

The Continuum begins

The reality is that the issues that started during creation or soon after due to trauma of birth infection and other impacting events have an identifiable pattern and will keep progressing unless intervention and rehabilitation occurs, which may be lifelong. What occurs is that the kids start showing up at the dentist's office according to a literature review on average between 3-7 years of age for preformed metal crowns[vii]. This is to correct dental cavities which will be blamed on poor oral hygiene, too much sugar or a bad diet by the dentist. Scant attention will be spent looking at the most likely causes, which include poor lip seal and mouth breathing (for a variety of reasons). At a similar period or perhaps slightly later the children will turn up at the speech therapists or the occupational therapist's office with speech language difficulties including lisps or oral hypersensitivity, apraxia, swallowing and feeding difficulties.

Then The children will appear at the orthodontic office starting between 12 and 15 years of age on average to have revision to the bite structure which has gone awry. The teeth will have been recognised to have been not right sooner, but the parent will have been told to wait till the child is older to intervene. Most often the focus is to improve the bite aesthetics and teeth meshing, and not improving airway or craniofacial structural development. It's interesting to note that compliance with orthodontic treatment appears better in younger subjects[viii], this is pertinent as a paper we will discuss suggests we have been intervening significantly later than optimal and that this has been known for 100 years.

Oxygen airway and the Brain

As we are all aware oxygen is of particular importance to the brain, thus the brain defends the airway to protect the nervous system along with heart pumping, especially at night when you can't consciously alter breathing rates and we must rely entirely on the Autonomic Nervous System (ANS) regulation for survival. Breathing is essential to life as you can't oxygenate easily without it occurring, therefore it is accorded a high propriety in the ANS and is given more resources to make sure it keeps occurring.

As you can see from the following picture the structure of the Cranium and airway, the airway is very narrow and can very easily be occluded by the tongue, especially if there is deviation of cranial development and function. The Tonsils, pharyngeal tissue of the soft palate can also occlude the airway.

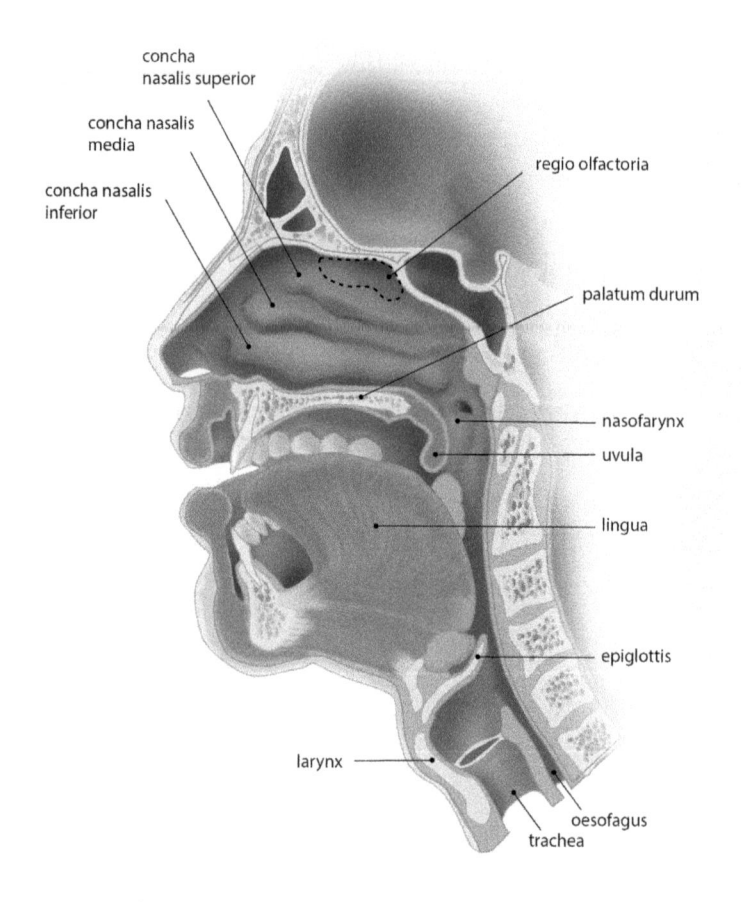

Image 1: A sagittal section of the nose, mouth, pharynx, and larynx. Notice how the tongue sits low in the oral cavity. At rest it should be touching the hard palette. Look at how narrow the airway is and the capacity for the tongue to occlude it, especially supine. https://anatomytool.org/content/slagter-drawing-head-and-neck-sagittal-section-latin-labels

My point is that we appear to overlook the importance of the oral/facial/cranial maldevelopment, mechanical dysfunction and ankyloglossia, their impacts on human health and neurocognitive development.

In medicine we tend to view and treat symptoms as discrete problems, and not as parts of a single or a greater problem that exists on a continuum. The Continuum of health suggests that very little is discrete, rather that if the function and structure that created symptoms are not corrected as a unit, and the human viewed as a whole, then further problems will continue to develop through life that can become deadly.

Think reflux, feeding issues, speech difficulties, orthodontic needs or snoring/apnoea, diabetes hypertension, strokes, and dementia. All these conditions can be associated with tongue tie and facial cranial dysfunction, missed in childhood. As we will see there is also a chicken versus the egg scenario as to whether neurological issues start the dysfunction or whether it starts in the oral structure. We will try to elucidate this in discussion of epigenetic dysfunction at about 5 weeks gestation.

So, let's dive into the continuum and see where the journey takes us.

Ankyloglossia/Tongue oral Restriction (Tongue Tie)

Ankyloglossia is the medical term for what is commonly known as tongue-tie. It is described as a congenital disorder with clinical signs of a low lingual frenulum, which limits movement of the tongue, and causes speaking and swallowing difficulties[ix]. It is considered an uncommon congenital oral anomaly that can cause difficulty with breast-feeding and later on speech articulation problems. We will see that it is surprisingly common, and the statistics don't do it justice.

Ankyloglossia is commonly classified according to Kotlow's classification system which has 4 classes.

Kotlow's tool is really considering the person's inability to pass the free tongue past the lower lip. The free tongue is defined as the length of the tongue from the insertion distance of the lingual frenulum to the tip of the tongue[x]. This classification tool is really only useful for assessment of anterior ties. Thus, I note that according to Nikki Mills; a New Zealand based expert on Tongue tie, the above tool neglects to classify posterior tongue ties or other variants, missing a lot of peoples issues and allowing health issues to develop long term. We need a better tool to suit the human population.

This discussion will try to explain the pathophysiology, classification, evaluation, and management of patients with ankyloglossia as well as cranial development dysfunction from preconception through to later adulthood. It highlights that Ankyloglossia is not a discrete occurrence of childhood but morphs into other issues seen at developmental stages or later phases of life such as orthodontic requirements and snoring/apnoea, which we have developed stand-alone treatment for without looking for the connecting thread. I will also try to highlight the role of the interprofessional team in treating and decreasing long term morbidity in patients with ankyloglossia[xi].

Ankyloglossia is an Oral fascial restriction which impacts significantly on the health and development of children. The awareness in infants has seen a spike in attention[xii] more towards breastfeeding and latch improvement than the massive impact on development, breathing, and sleep health. However, there is little mention of its impact on, or existence in the adult population, regardless of its impact on the function of the TMJ and cranium or disease progress in the adult population.

This is quite bizarre. If oral fascial restriction and craniofacial maldevelopment occurs in the infant, and is not intercepted and rehabilitated, then it will continue into adulthood potentially leading to developmental compensations away from optimal and health consequences.

Concerned parents are referred for tongue oral fascia releases for their newborns to help a child to breastfeed. But what about those of us who didn't get released earlier in life?

Adult oral facial restrictions are a much less talked about phenomena which we shall discuss along with the developmental impacts in children.

Posterior tongue tie

Posterior tongue tie, also known as a posterior ankyloglossia, is a form of tongue tie in which the tissue under the tongue is attached too far back in the mouth, restricting movement of the tongue. Here are some steps that may be taken to diagnose posterior tongue tie:

1. Physical examination: A healthcare professional will perform a physical examination of the tongue, looking for any abnormalities in the shape or movement of the tongue. They may also check for other signs of tongue tie, such as difficulty breastfeeding or latching onto a bottle.
2. Medical history: The healthcare professional may ask about the person's medical history, including any previous diagnoses or symptoms that may be related to tongue tie.
3. Imaging tests: In some cases, imaging tests such as an X-ray or ultrasound may be used to visualise the tongue and surrounding tissue.
4. Specialised assessment: Some healthcare professionals may use specialised assessments, such as the Lingual Frenulum Assessment Tool (LFAT) or the Ankyloglossia Functioning Score (AFS), to help diagnose posterior tongue tie.

Muscles of the Tongue

For everyone reading this book's ease of understanding I will describe the oral muscles and their action, if you have a firm grasp, please feel free to skip to the next section. The Muscles of the Tongue are categorised into the Extrinsic muscles and the Intrinsic Muscles. Understanding the action of the muscle and the tissue will help when imagining how they affect oral function, the skull development and movement, how the fascia connects to the substructures and the effects upon nerves and neurological development.

THE EXTRINSIC MUSCLES

Genioglossus muscle: This is a triangular looking Muscle which forms the bulk of the tongue and is a single muscle even if it is shown as having three parts. The genioglossus is essential for protrusion or to poke the tongue out and down the chin, using the muscle fibres that lie most anteriorly. The central part depresses the tongue, it draws the tip back and down.

This motion is what is commonly assessed for tongue tie using Kotlow's tool. If the patient can poke the tongue out and down the chin and retract it back into the mouth then tongue tie is ruled out or at least categorised for severity and a determination for capability to use a bottle is assessed, intervention is not the preferred action.

Palatoglossus muscle: This muscle elevates the posterior aspect of the tongue and is essential for the suck swallow and breath reflex to occur smoothly. It runs from the palate towards the tongue proper, and forms lateral arches situated at the back and lateral aspects of the throat. It is more closely associated with the soft palate both in situation and function, and it is not well assessed. The Palatoglossus works in opposition to the other muscles which are sublingual, pulling the tongue up and towards the posterior of the mouth cavity. Think sucking the tongue to the roof of the mouth and holding it there, this is the joy the Palatoglossus gives us. Thus, if it is tethered, short or dysfunctional such as poor tone, with low neurological activation, then it may be dominated by protrusion activities and never been seen as an issue.

Hypoglossus muscle: This is essential for tongue depression and retraction, is more like a sheet running from the body of the hyoid bone up towards the tongue. It depresses the tongue. Due to the angle of activation the Hypoglossus muscle can if short or tethered could be detrimental to the airway, leading to occlusion of the airway, especially if the person is sleeping on their back. As I will continue to mention, the brain must defend the airway, thus other muscles will be activated to pull the tongue up and out of the throat, if there is a discrepancy with this muscle or others in the mouth.

Styloglossus muscle: This muscle is essential for tongue retraction and elevation, the shortest and smallest of the three styloid muscles. It comes from the styloid process and goes towards the tongue. It retracts the tongue as it pulls back and elevates the posterior aspects of the tongue. Again, you can imagine its role in the essential suck, swallow, breathe reflex. Issues with this muscle and how it relates to the palatoglossus might make this quite difficult.

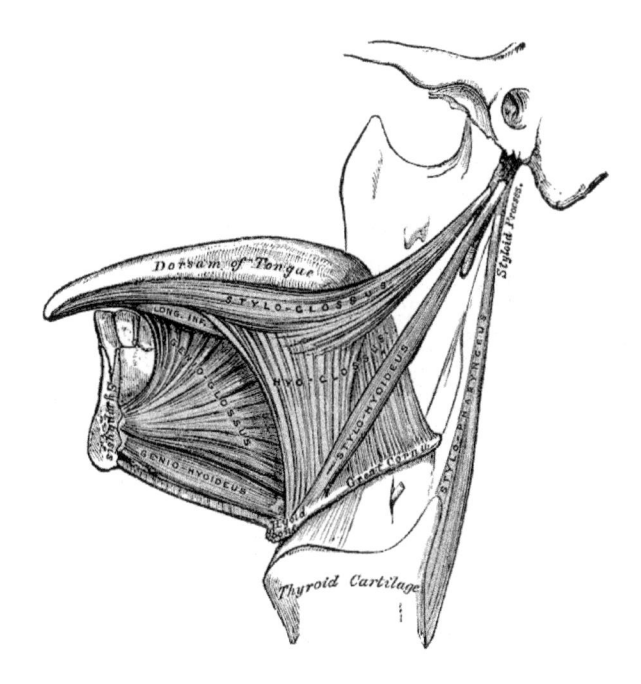

Image 2: Showing the Extrinsic muscles of the tongue and oral cavity including the styloglossus, genioglossus, Palatoglossus, Hypoglossus muscles. By Henry Vandyke Carter - Henry Gray (1918) Anatomy of the Human Body Bartleby.com: Gray's Anatomy, Plate 1019, PublicDomain, https://commons.wikimedia.org/w/index.php?curid=527364

THE INTRINSIC MUSCLES

- The intrinsic muscles are supplied by the hypoglossal nerve (CV XII), which enables the motor movement of the muscles. Notice there is a midline septum where both the intrinsic muscles lie on both sides of it.
- The superior longitudinal muscle runs along the length of the tongue towards the tip. Its function is to elevate, assist in retraction and bringing the tongue back into the oral cavity.

- The inferior longitudinal muscle lies deeper within the tongue and has a similar function in deviating the tongue to the side and pulls the tip of the tongue downwards inferiorly. This muscle also assists in the retraction of the tongue.
- The transverse muscle allows narrowing of the tongue, and as the name suggests, the muscle runs from the left to the right.
- Finally, there are the vertical muscle fibres which pull the tongue down towards the floor of the mouth.
- The Lingual nerve supplies many of the muscles of the tongue arises from the mandibular branch of the Trigeminal nerve, it is superficially located on the ventral surface of the tongue immediately below the fascia layer.

The Lingual Frenulum

Lingual frenulum is a lot more complex than we have been led to believe, it is the tissue of focus when we consider tongue tie in its most traditional sense. It is the connective string under the tongue that covers the nerves, blood vessels and muscles which connect the jaw to the skull, hyoid bone and provide many important functions essential for survival. It has multiple structures involved according to Dr Nikki mills, who has specialised in paediatric ankyloglossia investigations at the star ship children's hospital in Auckland New Zealand, and is a Maverick in the field, turning long held beliefs on their heads.

The lingual frenulum is not composed of connective tissue fibres that have an anteroposterior orientation nor is it a discrete cord or band as often described in literature. In contrast, the fascial fibres that form the frenulum have a basket-weave orientation as they cross the midline. This finding is supported by the histological study of adult cadavers from 1966 that reported a diagonal orientation of the collagenous fibres of the frenulum that crossed each other to form a scaffold-like framework (Fuchs, 1966). Consequently, the use of the terms such as cord, string, mast, or band to describe the lingual frenulum is misleading and should be discontinued. We suggest the structure of the lingual frenulum is described as a "**midline fold**." This term is inclusive of the morphological variations of mucosa, floor of mouth fascia and genioglossus fibres that may elevate into the fold that forms the frenulum with tongue elevation.[xiii]

To understand the Lingual frenulum, I have listed some important considerations both of its action and factors to bear in mind with any intervention surgery to reduce tongue tie.

The lingual frenulum is made of oral mucosa and is the fascia of the floor of the mouth, connected on top of the muscles. It is a dynamic 3-D structure that ranges on a spectrum, which causes a predicament for patients due to inter-examiner variability. We need a better tool for assessment, especially for posterior restriction and greater standardisation of what constitutes a need for surgery and rehabilitation versus which need neuromuscular rehabilitation and cranial adjustment alone. The frenulum is composed of a sheet of fascia and is not a discrete midline band of connective tissue, it suspends the floor of the mouth within the arc of the mandible and creates a balance between oral mobility and stability, not just for the tongue but also for jaw opening.

Care in any intervention is essential to avoid sensory nerve damage, this care is warranted especially when using hot lasers in any procedure for reduction as the risk for thermal damage to surrounding tissue and not just blunt trauma is possible.

There are direct bridges between the Ligurian nerve and the hypoglossal nerve which is the motor branch, this is the link between the environmental feedback to alter and contour intrinsic muscle shape of the dorsal tongue which is critical for intramural vacuum seal essential for milk extraction during feeding. But later for talking and expressive language, let alone intimate uses for the tongue.

We should always be aware that scar tissue formation occurs after all surgery as part of healing, however if the tongue is not activated by movement to elevate it, we risk reattachment and restriction of the motion we are trying to create by the intervention.

This means it is essential to provide active exercises to promote movement and growth in the appropriate direction, regardless of the age of the patient. This motion further enhances function by stimulating appropriate bone growth and development if early enough in the child's development.

It is important to note that if done early enough children's oral development will continue towards an uninterrupted baseline with normal function and strength, this is not usually the case in adults who have developed normal compensations for many years. These patients will need constant regular stimulus to maintain function and an occlusion-free airway, therefore finding meaningful activity such as playing a trumpet or using a Myo-nozzle to drink with for the long term is essential.

Reasons why tongue tie may not be diagnosed regularly

There are several reasons why tongue tie may not be diagnosed regularly:

1. **Lack of awareness:** Tongue tie is not a well-known condition, and many healthcare professionals may not

be aware of it or the potential impact it can have on a person's health. As a result, they may not consider it as a potential diagnosis.
2. **Difficulty identifying the condition:** Tongue tie can be difficult to identify, especially in infants and young children. The tissue under the tongue may be hard to see, and some cases of tongue tie may be very mild, making them difficult to detect.
3. **Limited screening:** Tongue tie is not routinely screened for in many healthcare settings, so it may not be detected unless it is specifically looked for, or parents have had a previous child with tongue tie and are pre warned about the condition.
4. **Misconceptions about the condition:** There are many misconceptions about tongue tie, including the belief that it is not a serious condition or that it will resolve on its own. This can lead to a lack of recognition and treatment of the condition, which sadly will lead to long term health consequences in many other areas.
5. **Drive to not intervene:** There is a prevalent hands-off response, a wait and see approach in health care which also then carries through to parental response. For the physician, this may stem from concern about being overly interventionist when unnecessary, however it may also stem from the concern about insurance costs and not being sued for making things worse.

Tongue tie, if not diagnosed appropriately in a child, it can lead to a range of consequences, including:

1. **Difficulty breastfeeding:** Tongue tie can make it difficult for an infant to breastfeed effectively, leading to

poor weight gain, a failure to thrive and other health problems.
2. **Speech delays:** Tongue tie can affect the development of speech and language skills in children, leading to delays in communication.
3. **Dental problems:** Tongue tie can cause problems with tooth alignment and jaw development, leading to dental problems in some cases.
4. **Difficulty swallowing:** Tongue tie can make it difficult for a child to swallow properly, leading to problems with feeding and malnutrition.
5. **Social and emotional issues:** Children with tongue tie may face social and emotional challenges due to difficulty communicating and participating in activities such as sports and games.

It is important to diagnose and treat tongue tie as early as possible to avoid these consequences and to improve the child's overall health and quality of life. It may be necessary to see multiple healthcare professionals to get a proper diagnosis. If you suspect that your child may have tongue tie, it is recommended to speak with a healthcare professional for a proper diagnosis and treatment plan.

Tongue tie problems in adults

For one reason or another, tongue-ties became a lost part of the paediatric assessment, both medical and dental. Up until the early twentieth century midwives were known to clip a newborn's tongue-tie at birth if spotted with a sharpened fingernail kept especially for this purpose. Retired paediatricians have reported a 'thrive or die' approach early in their careers. If newborns were found to have feeding or other issues, they were routinely checked for tongue tie as the most likely initial problem that could be resolved quickly.

We saw a decline in oral fascial restriction intervention in the second half of the 20th century along with a movement away from the practice of breastfeeding. This practice recommendation fortunately has taken a 180-degree U-turn and is back to breast is best.

The decline in tongue tie intervention appears to have been caused by or coincides with the rise of formula and bottle feeding, along with an increase in litigation and insurance concerns about intervention, which together, made diagnosing a tongue tie as a long-lost art.

The beginning of the 21st century has brought diagnosis of tongue tie back to life. With many papers published on oral facial development and the connection to postural change, behavioural and neuro-developmental issues.

Sadly, that means there are at least 2 and possibly 3 or 4 generations that had their tongue ties missed at birth with ongoing consequences, especially its impact on airway function as we will discuss. It's a large group of adults and could mean that **you** unknowingly have a tongue-tie.

Your tongue is such a crucial part of your body. The neuromuscular system is intertwined with the brain, the digestive system, the neck, spine, and teeth, as well as in spatial awareness, sound localisation and the capacity to emotively respond in an appropriate fashion.

The Tongue - our first sensory organ, motor unit, and so much more

The tongue is the first organ used and developed by the nervous system; it also is the first reflexogenic motor unit that we also learn to use volitionally. This is in its first role in feeding.

To understand human complexity consider swallowing itself involves 31 muscles, six cranial nerves and a few cervical and thoracic nerves.

In honesty though the tongue, mouth, and breastfeeding is about so much more than just a mouth latching onto the breast to take in milk.

It's about secure attachment as a human. The ability to connect with another person[xiv], primarily the mother. Which I believe is the basis for all human relationships.

We are literally hard wired for connection, security, and social emotional development from the mouth up and outwards. We come out of the womb, able to crawl up mums' belly to find our first sustenance, latching onto the breast, and we look up. We stare into mums' eyes, and we connect. Mum's face responds to us, and we develop, we start the interplay of neurological development that allows us to survive, it all begins with the mouth.

There is a massive connection between the neuromotor development of the mouth and the eye movements that influence many of our more adult actions. Problems with the discrete wiring of these systems start leaking early in childhood.

Consider a new-born baby, as it lays on its mother's tummy, it latches onto the breast, the eyes gaze up to stare at the mother's face, security, starting the nervous system development leading to postural reflex maturity (over time) as well as emotional maturity and self-security. Alteration in head position during feeding can alter posture development, leading to bone development change as well as emotional dysregulation[xv]. According to Rochat and Bullinger postural and emotional development is a major determinant of functional action in infancy and is based upon 3 observations, sucking, looking, and reaching.

Swallowing as an action is very much taken for granted and not thought about, we just do it, this is because it is a reflexogenic action that is hardwired to occur in our nervous system, as without being able to swallow you will die quite quickly soon after birth. It is an action that must occur, therefore if you can't perform it optimally due to an impediment, including poor neurological supply to or feedback from the muscles, structural alteration of the mouth or pharynx or perhaps an inability to breath, then a compensatory sub-optimal swallow will be devised by our very survival orientated brain, Think rule one above. Swallowing is however, very much affected by head positioning, both reflexogenic, and volitional posture, as well as cranial nerve function and cranial structural morphology all of which can alter function.

To give more colour to that statement let's look at a paper by Noirot and Algeria from 1982, which has been buried in the onslaught of publishing and has been largely forgotten. They demonstrated a difference in postural orientation between breastfed and bottle-fed babies. That's a huge finding, babies differentiate neurological function leading to postural structural differences early in life due to a difference in nutritive intake style!

The breast-fed baby will shift posture within the first 3 feeds to the direction of a human voice while the bottle-fed babies will orientate to the usual position of the caretaker.

This demonstrates that the collicular map is influencing postural control and development. The superior colliculus is part of the brainstem. It transforms sensory signals from many systems into the motor commands for orienting the person in space[xvi] and directing eye movements called saccades to selected targets[xvii]. Bullinger and Rochat demonstrated head orientation preference to feeding in new-borns helps drive survival. Their finding showed that head orientation altered sucking rate. Breastfed babies had a centre head sucking preference, while bottle fed babies had a right centre preference, but it appeared to correlate to past feeding preference by the caretaker of the child.

This again suggests that there is a large link between postural functional development, and midline structures with the innate preference centre with an up-eye position allowing the breast to fill the palette easily and drive "normal" cranial development as well as CNS reflex organic behaviour. Trauma during birth as well as environmental factors may alter normal development having consequences far beyond the mouth.

As a point the eye up saccade is connected to the vermis via the superior colliculus, it uses both sides of the cortex to control it and it provides stability cues to the midline trunk muscles for stability. Alteration of this function for any reason, lost wisdom, convenience, difficulty feeding etc will alter the normal pathways of eye neuronal circuitry in the brain/brainstem, leading to a change in the developmental pathways of the child and possibly compensation. Compensation is the rule of survival, see one above.

Further, this finding also suggests that traditional feeding styles of vertical child tummy to tummy position called Kangaroo care, will offer the best development posture for the child and that sideways hold and rugby hold may be aberrant to best development, postural as well as neuro/emotional capability.

As we can all appreciate, this is the pattern that is first demonstrated by the newborn, moments after birth, but is not encouraged or continued in western nations, so driven by convenience. Politeness of a lady not showing her breasts in public may also have driven the decline of what appears to be a better way of feeding for the child's development. Whatever the reason, it is not common today except in very traditional hunter gatherer type societies, even my new mothers struggle to get to grips with this idea when I encourage them in my practice. While there are no long-term studies evaluating the effect on our societies, I can't help but wonder what we are losing by not feeding for best development.

The study of feeding driving development is not new, but has fallen out of fashion for some reason, in 1998, Butterworth and Hopkins published a paper demonstrating that neonates open the mouth in anticipation of a hand brought towards the oral region, and that a drop of sugar on the tongue doubled the duration and frequency of manual contact with the mouth. The impact of this paper is huge, it clearly shows a causal link between eye hand postural position and tongue use, in a survive or die neuroplasticity model. These behaviours are driven by primitive reflexes and help drive development towards more adult neurological development. What I am alluding to is that if the neonate's posture is altered, we alter the developing functions of the neonate which appears to alter the CNS development.

Neonate Development

The neonate is born developmentally, very early compared to other mammals, with all needs being delivered by mother (and some fathers) and development being driven by reflexogenic behaviours and use of the neuromuscular system to cause the brain to grow and develop, enhancing survival. Thus, the importance of the dyad pair bonding effectively is so important to the healthy outcome of the child it almost can't be quantified, but we do see it in behaviours of other mammals such as sheep, where if the bonding doesn't occur in a specific time frame the mother will not accept the lamb and it will die without farmer intervention. Issues in the initial few days after birth can cause long term consequences for neuro-emotional development and according to the researchers of The Barker Hypothesis, it may create an alteration to the child's stress/threat set point for life and can increase health consequences such as diabetes, obesity, and heart disease. We will discuss The Barker Hypothesis further later on.

Breastfeeding effectively is essential to social emotional development for the whole life of the child, notwithstanding it strongly impacts the development of the structure and function of the skull and face and airway.

If the child is in a constant state of stress, from either internal body issues, feedback loops or from things in their environment, including mould, malnourishment, parental issues (predation) Their nervous system will wire pathways to view the world as threatening and react reflexogenically with an increase in vigilance, they will be in a constant state of reactivity to threat and alters sensitivity to catecholamines and epigenetically alters many other gene outcomes. Consider the old adage of "a good defence is a great offence. Kill it before it kills me and ask questions later", humans have this capacity hardwired in, the nurture concept is there to guide development away from this capacity.

The ability to build healthy relationships in later life appears to be based on effective connection to mother, to feel safe and secure and to use the cortical output of the mother for soothing and learning how to adapt to the environment, to consider and learn what is a threat and how best to respond, run, fight, or freeze.

Vagal Tone is a useful tool for determining stress state especially in infants. Psychologist and researcher Stephen Porges found that vagal tone can be used to monitor the neural control of the heart via the vagus as an index of homeostasis[xviii]. This has allowed us to assess the amount of environmental threat the infant may be under (also older humans) and consider its impact on the child's thriving or failure to. A paper by Fields[xix] and Diego investigating outcomes in mother child dyads demonstrated that in a sample separated by high and low anger, the high anger mothers had low vagal tone and high prenatal cortisol, epinephrine (noradrenaline) as well as low dopamine and serotonin levels, this was, in turn, mimicked by their neonates. This indicates the massive link between the infant learning how to view the world from mother, and the important impact that early interruption of smooth bonding, feeding, and environment has on our nervous system and its impact on long term health and well-being.

Low vagal activity was noted in prenatally depressed mothers as well as in prenatally angry and anxious mothers, and their infants, as well as in children with autism. These Researchers highlight relationships between vagal activity and the social behaviours of attentiveness, facial expressions, and vocalisations. Thus, the state of neurocognitive environment in the mother prior to during and after pregnancy, is mimicked and wires the state neurocognitive environment in the neonate.

This phenomenon is described in The Barker Hypothesis,[xx] The foetal origins hypothesis and combines several key ideas about early impact on human health long after the initial threat has left the infant.

First, the effects of foetal conditions are persistent. Second, the health effects can remain latent for many years – for example heart disease does not typically emerge as a problem until middle age. Third, the hypothesised effects reflect a specific biological mechanism of foetal "programming," possibly through effects of the environment on the epigenome, which are just beginning to be understood. The epigenome can be conceived of as a series of switches that cause various parts of the genome to be expressed – or not. This is important when we consider possible causes of tongue tie or craniofacial dysfunction developing from the middle of the pregnancy leading to ongoing airway and cognitive change.

Development: Function drives form

The foetus begins moving its tongue at about 12.5 weeks[xxi] of gestation and by week 18[xxii] (almost halfway through pregnancy) the foetus has developed a swallow mechanism. If this movement is not normal/easy, such as due to tethering and restriction in the tissues of the oral mucosa, then the child will start to develop compensatory mechanisms of use.

Consider the earliness of the tongue structural and reflexogenic development in life. This means that the infant has had plenty of time practising using a mechanism that is very likely less efficient, wiring it into the CNS before breast feeding even has occurred.

Consider then, that a lot of breastfeeding after birth may be an abnormal compensatory mechanism when compared to optimal and expected action, leading to alteration of the muscle development of the face and cranium, affecting how the structure develops. A new mother will not know if it is less efficient as she could not observe the foetus's development nor has any idea of what perfect latch and feeding might feel like, thus development can continue off in an aberrant developmental trajectory.

Ultimately compensatory movement and use leads to changes in how the child experiences and interacts with the world, and likely development of symptoms. This can show up as failure to thrive, oral sensitivity, colic, positing, spilling of milk, drooling, picky eating, speech language issues (as seen by a speech therapist, or OT), fragmented sleep, anxious behaviour as well as orthodontic issues so common in the society and many other issues.

46 • SCOTT WUSTENBERG

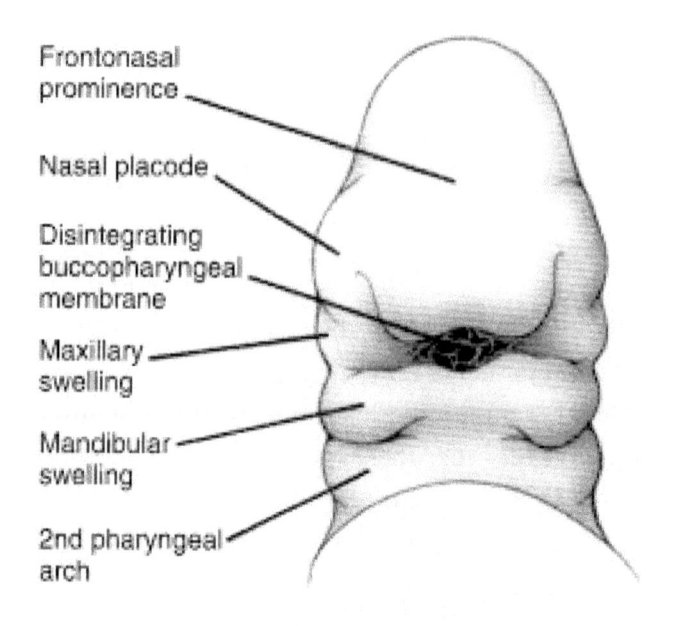

Frontonasal prominence
Nasal placode
Disintegrating buccopharyngeal membrane
Maxillary swelling
Mandibular swelling
2nd pharyngeal arch

5th week

Image 3: The above image shows the origin of the human face and mouth and tongue. The face develops from five primordia that appear in the fourth week: the frontonasal prominence, the two maxillary swellings, and the two mandibular swellings. The buccopharyngeal membrane breaks down to form the opening to the oral cavity. The notochord activates the fear paralysis reflex at week five integrating into the facial, throat and trunk structure, which appears to alter vagal tone long term, especially if aberration of normal function happens. http://www.columbia.edu/itc/hs/medical/humandev/2004/Chapt11-FacialPalatalDev.pdf

What is normal?

I SHALL USE the term normal to describe a optimal expected development that is similar in all humans, I accept that no one ever develops exactly the same, that is impossible, however "Normal" facial muscle activation in a regular symmetrical movement pattern, including the lips, and tongue, will lead to normal oral facial movement, think suck swallow breath reflex, which leads onto normal cranial movement and structural growth. Poor movement, or a lack of it can cause a lack of growth such as underdeveloped jaws, a lack of tone, seen in kids with excessive dribbling and drooling or a narrow face and in extreme cases plagiocephaly. The suck swallow breathe reflex is in action by about week 32 of the pregnancy. This is essential for "normal" breast feeding to occur with ease and no compensation and given that function drives form, alteration in this reflex can contribute to structural alteration.

It can't be overstated how important normal motion is for brain and cognition development which is led by primitive reflexes and the hard wired reflexogenic capacity built into the brainstem and spinal cord. It's noted in neuroscience research that if you can't make a specific motor pattern on your face, you can't easily understand the emotion[xxiii] it pertains too. It is worth considering therefore the concepts of children with low tone or restriction of facial muscles and the difficulty these children have. Trying to develop emotional maturity, if you can't make the pattern how can you understand it or express it.

Thus, the deep front line of the body, which can be viewed as the fascia connections and midline structures including hip and shoulder girdle muscles, eyes, lips, tongue, abdominal muscles, and the hearing complex are essential for normal development of the neonate posture towards adult growth. These functions provide the ability to locate oneself in space as well as move and locomote, for survival and later on for fun, they also give the capacity to calm and later will go on to develop and integrate volitional control of higher thinking centres in the CNS. Normal movement is essential for healthy development cognitively and posturally and the possibility of life free of disease.

Developmental Form: The evidence for maldevelopment

In this section I will discuss some of the literature about epigenetics and the research that has gone into our understanding of facial structural development and what makes us function. Lots of the work is done on animal models and in labs and has been extrapolated to apply to humans, I believe the story I have put together is compelling and should be investigated further so we can have better long-term health outcomes.

Where we shall start is looking at the results of experiments performed in zebrafish,[xxiv] which demonstrate that cerebrospinal fluid (CSF) flow[xxv] in the skull and spine effects facial development of the embryos and can lead to postural aberration and scoliosis. The CSF movement in the spinal system contributes to long term healthy functional outcomes in the adult animal or negative ones. The experiments deduced that this is partially related to the retinoic acid carrying protein (RAR), and problems with it.

This protein carries vitamin A and precursors around the CSF and is associated with alteration in CSF flow and embryonic cell survival, thus low maternal vitamin A or precursors may have a negative impact on skeletal development during pregnancy, as does excessive levels of free Retinoic acid in the plasma.[xxvi] This scenario leads to bone resorption and issues with structural fragility.

Work done by Kennedy and Dickinson in 2012 revealed that inhibition of retinoic acid signalling during facial specification in Xenopus embryos results in median clefts in the primary palate[xxvii] which is related to tongue tie.

Retinoic acid Receptor (RAR) inhibition resulted in significantly reduced intercanthal distance, reflecting a narrower midface, and an increased face height, reflecting changes in brain position as well as an alteration in sinus structure adding to the possibility of airflow change.

In addition, these embryos had a smaller mouth angle, and significantly increased midline mouth height[xxviii]. This is pretty exciting stuff as it shows nutrients have critical effects on development and things that are easy to alter in diet to alter outcomes. It raises questions about nutrition screening in young women before pregnancy, food fortification and whether the drive to consume high amounts of plant-based beta carotene versus consumption of animal-based Vitamin A is having positive or negative impacts on the paediatric development, especially as we know they have SNP for conversion of beta-carotene to Vitamin A which affect availability to the organism. This work also critically demonstrates structural alteration in our offspring's cranial structure, that might affect outcomes in later life.

We further know that environmental factors such as ethanol in the bloodstream, similar to levels occurring from binge drinking can alter skeletal development in mouse and zebrafish models leading to scoliosis and cleft palate. This raises some interesting questions about critical timing of exposure and the dose of the toxin as it relates to conditions such as foetal alcohol syndrome, and towards our oral facial structural maldevelopment issues, which may cause tongue tie and narrow palates. Perhaps there are sublevels of maldevelopment that occur when dosed earlier or at a lower amount which alters skeletal outcomes, which impacts CNS development.

Problematically at the 4-6 week mark of gestation many women may not be aware of being pregnant and thus may not be aware of inducing a problem in the child's post-partum life, with what can ostensibly be considered "normal" or at least common behaviour.

Clearly, we have some society level discussions to come if we want to change health outcomes in our race.

Nutrition links to Ankyloglossia and facial development issues

Epigenetics refers to the study of changes in gene expression or function that do not involve changes to the underlying DNA sequence. These changes can be influenced by a variety of factors, including environmental exposures, diet, and certain genetic mutations. Consider it the silencing or the activation of an outcome, from the gene which will influence our growth and behaviour. Epigenetics can alter the shape and form of expressed proteins, increasing the speed of a function or slowing it down. It may even silence its expression altogether.

Epigenetic SNP's Associated with Oral function Change

There is evidence to suggest that epigenetic changes may be involved in the development of tongue tie. For example, a study published in the Journal of Clinical and Experimental Dentistry found that epigenetic changes in the promoter region of the Transforming growth factor beta-3 (TGFB3) gene may play a role in the development of tongue tie. TGFB3 is a protein that in humans is encoded by the TGFB3 gene. It is a type of protein, known as a cytokine, which is involved in cell differentiation, embryogenesis, and development. Variance in the gene may cause more fibrous tissue growth and a lack of apoptosis during development, this could be a pathway creating the tension and alteration of the lingual frenulum.

It's highly likely that you may have heard of the next SNP, it has been given an almost mythical status in health and disease, especially in the Autism field, and integrative medicine. It is capable of effecting many areas, but many patients after diagnosis tend to blame it for all of their ills which is unlikely to be the case. Please keep in mind: All genes where normal variant or a SNP version code information, however that information is completely inert unless acted upon by an outside force a stimulus trigger. It does not do anything by itself. Think of it in the same way as a bottle of water on a bench with dehydrating person in front of it. The bottle can't do anything until the person picks it up and takes the cap off it, and drinks.

This analogy is very pertinent as to how Methylenetetrahydrofolate reductase (MTHFR) works in the body. MTHFR is an enzyme that plays a key role in the metabolism of folate, a B vitamin that is important for many bodily functions. In nature folate, and all B vitamins occur in an inactive state, like the aforementioned Bottle of water. The enzyme must act upon the folate and change its structure to allow it to be used in metabolism, just like the hand taking the cap off the bottle to make the water accessible, it acts in some way like a rate limiting step in methylation cycle reactions.

MTHFR gene mutations, more accurately called Single Nucleotide Polymorphisms (SNP's) can cause a range of health problems, including an increased risk of birth defects, cardiovascular disease, and certain types of cancer. The SNP itself can change the speed and efficiency of action of the protein/enzyme on its target. It could make it act faster increasing the amount of activated Folate or more commonly it makes it run slower, decreasing the amount of folinic acid produced. Please keep in mind methylation and frankly most metabolic processes we really need a goldilocks moment, meaning the speed and efficiency should be "Just Right", neither too fast or too slow, as toxic by-products may be produced or other parts of the cycle can be impeded.

There is evidence to suggest that there is a link between MTHFR gene mutations and tongue tie. A few studies have found an increased prevalence of MTHFR gene mutations in people with tongue tie and oral fascial restrictions in the midline, although the exact nature of the link is not yet fully understood.

As a public service announcement: It's important to note that tongue tie can have many different causes, and MTHFR gene mutations are just one possible factor. If you are concerned about a potential link between MTHFR and tongue tie, it is recommended to speak with a healthcare professional for a proper diagnosis and treatment plan.

DHFR (Dihydrofolate reductase) along with MTHFR and folic acid has been implicated in the development of ankyloglossia[xxix]. As an aside DHFR and MTHFR are enzymes that convert inactive folate found in food from the diet to an active version that the body can use in its cycles to make metabolism including neurotransmitter production occur. No B vitamins in nature are in the active or Methylated form, they all require enzymatic activation, and go through several steps to get to a usable state.

First Principles • 53

Folate metabolism | **Carbon metabolism**

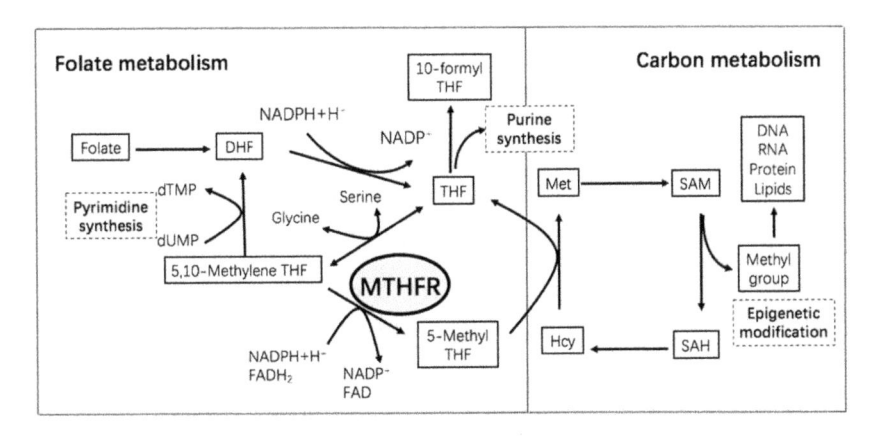

Image 4: Wan, L., Li, Y., Zhang, Z. *et al.* Methylenetetrahydrofolate reductase and psychiatric diseases. *Transl Psychiatry* **8**, 242 (2018). https://doi.org/10.1038/s41398-018-0276-6 [xxx]

In a paper by Amitai et al[xxxi], on "preconception care and folic acid", it was hypothesised that too much folic acid is problematic for the normal development of the foetus, leading to tighter midline structures and this being the cause of ankyloglossia. While I don't agree in total with this concept especially due to the results of other work, I've studied there is merit in the concept. Importantly, we can extrapolate from their study the concept that, "if we disturb the expression of genes essential for development due to teratological input at a critical developmental phase we can have long reaching consequences" in my opinion it can cause changes to cranial development, ossification, and outcomes for breathing after birth, as well as to emotional regulation and other issues.

If we change the shape of the skull, including the nasal structure, sinuses, the palette length or shape, the jaw rami length or shape, then we will alter the position and posture of the tongue in the mouth, we may also alter the ability to breathe through the nose and narrow the airway. This is also a vice versa scenario. Change to the tongue posture and function impedes the structural growth of the bones they contact.

This is demonstrated in work by Kennedy and Dickenson, that DHFR deficiency, specifically during early head and facial development causes a narrower midface and malformed mouth shape, due to loss of jaw muscle and cartilage elements. This is consistent with reported effects in mammals where folate deficiencies or mutations to major pathway components can also result in craniofacial defects and smaller head size[xxxii].

Folate and its active downstream components are essential for effective apoptosis, loss of folate metabolism for any reason, was demonstrated to alter appropriate facial/cranial development leading to small face and jaw development. This is consistent with reports in other vertebrates where defects in folate metabolism also resulted in increased apoptosis during development. DHFR inhibition induced apoptosis is in part due to increased DNA damage. Cells with defective folate metabolism would fail to generate sufficient thymidine, which can lead to genomic instability of the DNA. This can also be due to oxidative stress generated when the folate pathway is abrogated it can cause DNA damage-induced cell death[xxxiii].

Interestingly, it appears DNA damage could be a conserved effect of DHFR deficiency, Brooklyn et al found that children with folic acid deficiencies have increased levels of DNA damage in the palate[xxxiv], supporting this thought process.

DHFR deficient cells localised to regions of the face that correlated well with shape changes that have been identified in the midface by geometric morphometrics, that being a fancy way of saying we. Measured the shape change in the cellular structure in the face of the kids. In addition, developmental genes important for cartilage and muscle differentiation such as RAR's (retinoic acid receptors), FGFS (fibroblast growth factor gene) and WNTS (Wingless-related integration site gene) are expressed in the midface region, where there are abundant apoptotic cells.

Defects in folic acid metabolism during facial development results in a significant loss of cells expressing the genes (including WNTS, and FGFS) which are essential for facial structure formation, profoundly affecting the shape and size of the face[xxxv] of the developing foetus, leading to maldevelopment of the face in the child after birth and ongoing consequences in life.

Other epigenetic changes that have been linked to tongue tie include changes in DNA methylation issues, RBP (RNA-binding protein) changes and histone modification. A histone is a highly basic protein abundant in lysine and arginine amino acid residues that are found in the eukaryotic cell nuclei. They act as spools around which DNA winds to create the structural units called nucleosomes to help our genes hold structure and be appropriately packed in nucleus and allow appropriate reading of the genes. The exact nature of these links and the mechanisms by which they may influence the development of tongue tie are not yet fully understood. However, if the histone is misshapen due to modification and inappropriate tagging of the DNA, then the gene may be read out of sequence leading to the protein structure they make being misfolded and the structure they create to be dysfunctional as a result. The bonds don't pull in the right place to make the 3-dimensional geometric structure hold its shape. It may be too rigid to work or too floppy as possibilities. Therefore, the function changes, like a protein that is meant to act as a lock for a cellular key, if it is too rigid it may not shape change to fit the key and the machinery fails to work.

It's important to note that tongue tie can have many different causes, and epigenetic changes are just one possible factor. If you are concerned about a potential link between epigenetic changes and tongue tie, it is recommended to speak with a healthcare professional for a proper diagnosis and treatment plan.

There are several nutritional deficiencies that may increase the risk of maxillary hypoplasia, also known as a narrow palate or narrow maxilla. These include:

1. **Folic acid deficiency:** Folic acid is a B vitamin that is important for normal growth and development, including the development of the palate. A deficiency of folic acid during pregnancy or early childhood may increase the risk of maxillary hypoplasia.
2. **Vitamin A deficiency:** Vitamin A is important for the proper functioning of the immune system and the development of the palate. A deficiency of vitamin A during pregnancy or early childhood may increase the risk of maxillary hypoplasia.
3. **Iron deficiency:** Iron is important for the production of red blood cells and the proper functioning of the immune system. A deficiency of iron during pregnancy or early childhood may increase the risk of maxillary hypoplasia.
4. **Protein deficiency:** Protein is important for the growth and repair of tissues, including the palate. A deficiency of protein during pregnancy or early childhood may increase the risk of maxillary hypoplasia.

It's important to note that these are just a few examples of the nutritional deficiencies that may increase the risk of maxillary hypoplasia. If you are concerned about the potential impact of nutritional deficiencies on your health or the health of your child, it is recommended to speak with a healthcare professional for a proper diagnosis and treatment plan.

Palette Hypoplasia - consequences and concerns

A narrow palate, also known as a narrow maxilla or maxillary hypoplasia, refers to a condition in which the roof of the mouth (palate) is smaller than normal. A narrow palate can lead to a range of health problems, including:

1. **Breathing problems:** A narrow palate can contribute to breathing problems, such as sleep apnoea, due to the reduced size of the airway.
2. **Dental problems:** A narrow palate can cause problems with tooth alignment and jaw development, leading to dental problems in some cases.
3. **Speech and language delays:** A narrow palate can affect the development of speech and language skills in children, leading to delays in communication.
4. **Eating difficulties**: A narrow palate can make it difficult for a person to eat and swallow properly, leading to problems with feeding and malnutrition.
5. **Social and emotional issues:** People with a narrow palate may face social and emotional challenges due to difficulty communicating and participating in activities such as sports and games.

Facial Malformations and Hypoplasia

From the above we can see that there is a lot of dysfunctions that can occur in cranial and midline development way beyond just ankyloglossia, clefts while less common give greater visual awareness of the midline dysfunction There are different types of clefts including lip and cleft palate that can be seen clinically. Complete clefts indicate the maximum degree of cleft of any type (e.g., a complete cleft of the secondary palate, a complete cleft of lip, alveolar process and primary palate, or a combination of these two). Incomplete clefts are found when some merging or fusion has taken place during development. Clefts may be unilateral or bilateral as seen in Images 5 and 6 below.

The important thing to remember clinically is that each site where merging or fusion occurs during development of face and palate is a potential site for a facial/palatal cleft[xxxvi].

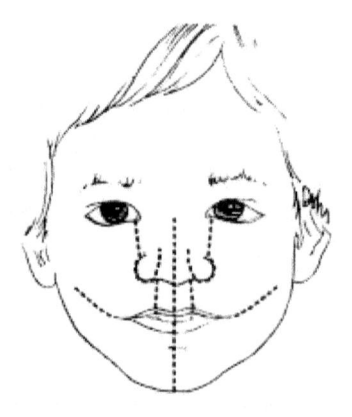

Image 5: In this diagram of a face, the broken lines indicate the possible locations of facial clefts. The areas between the broken lines correspond with the areas formed by the original facial processes. http://www.columbia.edu/itc/hs/medical/humandev/2004/Chapt11-FacialPalatalDev.pdf

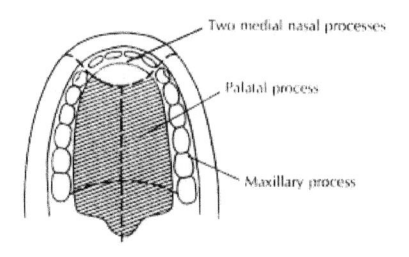

Image 6: A diagram of the hard and soft palates, as they appear viewed from below. The area of the front teeth corresponds with the primitive palate, formed largely by the two medial nasal processes. The shaded part of the palate (part of the hard palate in front, and the soft palate in the back) is formed by the two palatal processes, which come together and fuse in the midline. Clefts are possible at all "seams" between the medial nasal processes and the palatal processes and in the midline between the two palatal processes. http://www.columbia.edu/itc/hs/medical/humandev/2004/Chapt11-FacialPalatalDev.pdf

AS I PREVIOUSLY MENTIONED, the midline structures and especially how important the role of the mesio-palatine suture is in the nasomaxillary complex growth cannot be overstated. Deviation of cartilaginous cell migration to this area alters the complex ossification process of the facial structures, leading to long term growth alteration in structure and function. which compromises human development.

Let's consider the origin of craniofacial bone development. The skull bones must grow in a coordinated, three-dimensional manner to coalesce and form the head and face. Mammalian skull bones have a dual embryonic origin from cranial neural crest cells and paraxial mesoderm and ossify through intramembranous ossification. The bones of the cranium which cover the brain, are derived from the supraorbital arch (SOA) region mesenchyme. The SOA is the site of frontal and parietal bone morphogenesis and the primary centre of ossification.[xxxvii] Unlike trunk neural crest cells that migrate to relatively deep levels of the body forming organ tissue, the cranial neural crest cells migrate superficially. Neural crest cells emerging in the cranial region are distinct from those in trunk because they will give rise to osteoblasts and chondrocytes in addition to other cell types that trunk neural crest cells can differentiate into.[xxxviii]

Cartilage is a connective tissue made of chondrocytes embedded in a collagen-rich matrix (particularly type II collagen), associated with proteoglycans in hyaline cartilage that strengthen it, as well as elastin (depending on the type of cartilage). Hyaline cartilage is the forerunner to skeletal bones in the foetus, and endochondral ossification is the process leading to formation of the nasomaxillary complex.

The Chondrocranium develops in the second month of gestation and is reliant on nutritional availability of the maternal environment, this is not genetics, this is epigenetic. If mum is deficient in bone development nutrients such as, Vitamin A, folate, vitamin D, and K2 there will be inhibition of the cranial base growth, facial structure alteration and midline structural issues. The nutritional supply is deeply affected by activation of the fear paralysis reflex which we will discuss later. But for now, please be aware that it partitions nutrient, blood supply and resources towards the mother's system when environmental threat occurs, to enhance mother and child's survival. This reflex should turn off and return supply after immediate danger has passed. The problem is that a lot of environmental stress in the modern world is chronic as is the epidemic of anxiety which can also active the reflex.

The end result is malnourishment and maldevelopment, and an imprinting on the epigenome far away from optimal.

Of special interest is the exposure of the maternal environment to chemicals which can activate the fear paralysis reflex and cause blood supply partitioning. Some of these chemicals however have been shown to go through the maternal placental barrier and alter the foetus in potentially unfavourable ways. Chemicals such as methotrexate could have long reaching consequences. It is known to inhibit folate, while electric cigarette chemicals, nicotine, and artificial food like flavours such as vanillin can inhibit the retinoic acid receptor and act as an antagonist[xxxix].

That candy bar or quick hit that is meant to be safe, may actually cause unintended events to occur before you're aware you're pregnant. Further investigation down this path is warranted, given the rise in orofacial dysfunction in society, and the increase in vaping.

Currently the Australian government does monitor some nutritional statuses such as Folate, but it does not appear to monitor the degree of Vitamin A intake or deficiency[xl] in men or women (especially women in this case), and the official data available for public study is 10 years out of date. Looking at this data and their official interpretation, suggests that childbearing women all have adequate Folate levels. From their 2011 report, "The vast majority of women of childbearing age had sufficient folate levels in 2011–12. Folate is known to be important for preventing neural tube defects (NTDs) in developing babies, most notably spina bifida. Overall, they continue, "less than 1% of women aged 16–44 years had red cell folate levels in the at-risk range for NTDs" (less than 906 nmol/L)"[xli].

Let's consider this from a different viewpoint, as the literature may be obscuring the full truth.

Their report is at odds with the research literature for tongue tie and orthodontics. "The incidence of ankyloglossia in the new-born well-baby population is 4.8%"[xlii]. From our previous discussion we know that aberration in folate metabolism can lead to tongue tie.

"The mean prevalence of Angle Class I, Class II and Class III malocclusion was 51.9% (SD 20.7), 23.8% (SD 14.6) and 6.5% (SD 6.5), respectively. The prevalence of anterior crossbite, posterior crossbite and crossbite with functional shift was 7.8% (SD 6.5), 9.0% (SD 7.34) and 12.2% (SD 7.8), respectively. The prevalence of hypodontia and hyperdontia were reported to be 6.8% (SD 4.2) and 1.8% (SD 1.3), respectively[xliii]. Our discussion above proves conclusively that folate issues alone cause significant facial alteration leading to tongue tie and orthodontic end points, thus when the data shows a 5% ankyloglossia rate (1999) and a minimum of 12% structural shift in facial development requiring orthodontics, then perhaps the figure of less than 1% of childbearing women having folate deficiency may need review?

Mouth Breathing and Tonsils Activates the Immune System and Affects the Biome.

Cranio- facial growth is extremely important for all human outcomes. The lower portion of the face is purposely underdeveloped at birth to allow the baby to exit the birth canal with ease. Use and movement of the jaws and facial muscle including the tongue allow the bone structure to develop to more appropriate size in the first few years of life and resembles the adult face structure by three to four years of age.

Habitual behaviours of posturing with the tongue have a number of important benefits to the postural system but if done in a compensatory fashion can also lead to negative consequences. Ideally tongue position should be up and forward on the palette, and not retruded into the nasopharyngeal space.

First Principles • 63

A large enough and appropriately shaped nasopharyngeal space will facilitate nasal vs. mouth breathing. Nasal breathing is essential for health and serves several functions not given by mouth breathing. Breathing through the sinuses warms and humidifies the air. Filtration of the air of particulate matter is provided by the nasal hair as well as the mucous lining the airway before passing through the adenoids for further cleaning. The final step before entering the lungs is the tonsils. This process maximises Oxygen to carbon dioxide exchange while facilitating nitric oxide production in the sinuses. NO2 stimulates vasodilation in the lungs for efficient gas diffusion across the wall; it also acts as a potent antibacterial and antiviral agent.

Mouth breathing[xliv] requires that the tonsils should do all of this work. Mouth Breathing commonly leads to enlargement and inflammation of the tonsils, called tonsillitis.

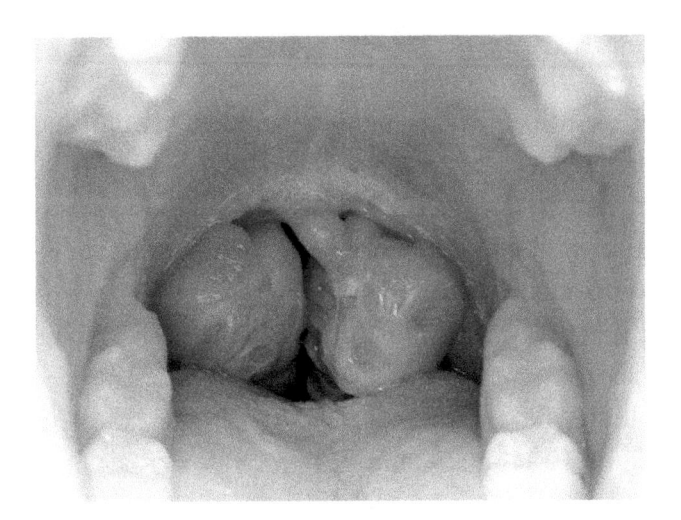

Image 7: The above indicates significant tonsillitis and encroachment of the tonsils into the airspace. Photo courtesy of: Paediatrics and Child Health Division of The Royal Australasian College of Physicians and The Australian Society of Otolaryngology, Head and Neck Surgery. [xlv]

INFECTIOUS TONSILLITIS IS a common issue in both children and adults and is frequently treated with antibiotics. In the UK recurrent sore throat/tonsilitis has an incidence of 100 per 1000 population per year. 10 percent of the population. Acute tonsillitis is more common in childhood but continues in mouth breathing adults. Common bacterial pathogens include beta-haemolytic and other streptococci. Bacteria are cultured from only a minority of people with tonsillitis, while the role of virus's play is uncertain. In tonsillitis associated with infectious mononucleosis, the most common infective agent is the Epstein-Barr virus (present in 50% of children and 90% of adults with the condition). Cytomegalovirus infection may also result in the clinical picture of infectious mononucleosis, and the differential diagnosis also includes toxoplasmosis, HIV, hepatitis A, and rubella[xlvi]. Antibiotics often have unintended consequences and may be unnecessary in most tonsillitis cases[xlvii]. The real thing to consider is that if you bypass all the nasal machinery for cleaning the air intake, then the tonsils must do the work. They will filter dust debris and particulate matter including mould and mould spores, cockroach dander, and a vanity of environmental toxins. This constant barrage activates the lymphatics and drives upregulation of the immune response creating a doom loop. The more activation due to mouth breathing the larger the tonsils become the more occlusion if the airway the more difficult it is to breath nasally, leading to more mouth breathing, snoring, hypopneas further immune activation, cytokine production, enlargement of the tonsils and so on. This loop has been shown to have significant neurological developmental consequences for increased stress and even is postulated to lead to schizophrenia development[xlviii].

As far back as 1945 it was being discussed that antibiotics may not be the panacea and end up having impacts on future health.

According to Blaser A variety of evidence indicates that the risks appear greatest for young children.[xlix] He also noted that the perinatal period through the first 2 years of life is the time when per capita antibiotic usage is most intensive. Blaser Raises the hypothesis that antibiotic courses may lead to species loss, especially for taxa that were low in number, but may have important metabolic functions. The problem would be most important for taxa with unique functions, because we each inherit much of our microbiome from our mother. A further hypothesis is that environmental impacts on the microbiome (including antibiotic and dietary exposures) are cumulative across generations. The implications are substantial. Once a bacteria population is gone from the mother's biome, she cannot hand it on to her offspring, thus it is lost to the child[l]. As you can see mouth breathing and oral dysfunction has fingers into so many areas of development and long-term health.

Mouth Posture Loops

Posturing with the mouth open lowers and retrudes the tongue, mandible, and hyoid bone. This can occlude the oropharyngeal airway space resulting in compensatory posterior cranial rotation to further open the airway. As a result of this re-posturing to level the point of fixation of the ocular plane due to the upper cervical and cranial base extension, the neck must assume a more forward position with reduced cervical lordosis.[li]. The mandibular and tongue retrusion that occurs with a mouth breathing posture are associated with the hyoid moving posteriorly and inferiorly which can further occlude the already narrow airway. Forward head posture helps to restore the hyoid position and further increase airway patency[lii].

Mouth breathing also facilitates increased accessory muscle breathing use and is associated with shoulder tension and muscle balance asymmetries. Mouth breathing is correlated to decreased nocturnal genioglossus, tensor palatine, upper airway dilator, and intercostal activity which can facilitate airway obstruction[liii]. The muscle imbalance produced by these changes may contribute to the mechanical disadvantage of the diaphragm and the increased effort of the accessory muscles of inspiration[liv]. Furthermore, forward head posture lengthens and narrows the airway making it more prone to collapse during inspiration thus encouraging hypopnea/apnoea behaviours[lv]. Confirming this loop, Ulhig et al found that: "Respiratory and postural adaptations increased the chances of individuals persisting with mouth breathing. Additionally, these adaptations could be associated with mouth breathers' self-perceived quality of life"[lvi]. Veron et al. found that the forward head posture that mouth breathers compensate with facilitates air to enter the mouth which can lead to a deterioration of the pulmonary function. In the long run, the hyperactivity of the neck muscles may be associated with cervical changes that, as a result, can cause temporomandibular disorders (TMD) and spine cervical disorders. Considering all these aspects, a cycle seems to be established where mouth breathing alters the respiratory function and mechanics and produces postural compensations, which in turn perpetuate the respiratory changes[lvii].

Cranial Development

A significantly important point is that no part of the face is developmentally independent after birth of any other part of the face/cranium. The arch development which is driven by tongue movement will affect the airway development and nasal sinuses, which effects eye position and head shape as well as jaw shape, and the shape of the cranial vault housing the brain.

The cranial base is a multifunctional bony platform within the core of the cranium, spanning rostral to caudal ends. This structure provides support for the brain and skull vault above, serves as a link between the head and the vertebral column below, and seamlessly integrates with the facial skeleton at its rostral end. Unique from most of the cranial skeleton, the cranial base develops from a cartilage intermediate the chondrocranium through the process of endochondral ossification. Owing to the intimate association of the cranial base with nearly all aspects of the head, congenital birth defects impacting these structures often coincide with anomalies of the cranial base[lviii].

At its most simple the cranial base provides the platform for facial as well as brain development.

It is essential for airway development and comprises the ossification centres of the sphenobasilar bone, disturbance to these centres could alter airway development as well as cranial nerve function as most cranial nerves come out through this bone.

As I've already noted, the chondrocranium develops in the second month of gestation and its healthy progress is reliant on nutritional status, placental availability to the maternal circulation, epigenetic switching, which may cause disruption to the cranial base bone growth and neurological reflex input to operate in an optimal sequence. Deficiencies in nutrients that help bone development including vitamin D, K2, vitamin A, magnesium or vitamin E may be catastrophic or mild, sadly we do not have enough evidence to determine effect from these building block changes.

Lots of cranial growth occurs during pregnancy, which is directly impacted by partition of nutrients by the gut lining as well by the placenta.

If malnourishment in the 2 years prior to pregnancy occurs in the mother due to environmental stresses, mal-digestion or bad diet occurs this will alter cranial development in the offspring (Barker hypothesis) along with alterations in health and well-being down to the third generation.

Nutrition will affect the sphenoid size and the size of the face. The Precursors of the sphenoid sinus are demonstrable in the fourth month of gestation as posterior recesses of the early nasal cavity which extend into the adjacent cartilage. The walls of the chambers which house these recesses are known as the ossicles of Bertin. The ossicles begin to ossify in the fifth month of gestation but do not fuse with the sphenoid bone proper until about the fourth year of life. Pneumatization of the sphenoid bone proper does not start until this osseous union is accomplished. At birth the primordial sinus cavities may be several millimetres in diameter. By the fourth or fifth year they have usually grown sufficiently to establish close relationship with important adjacent structures[lix]. However, these sinus structures can be consequentially altered by mouth breathing, and sinus infection, notwithstanding malnourishment or orthodontic and dental intervention.

The Palette

The current view in the literature, is that infants with obstructive sleep apnoea who are of normal weight and size, can considered to have a disorder of oral-facial growth". This has been observed specifically in infants who had a normal hard palate and maxilla at birth, but by their 6-month-old follow-up visit they had developed an abnormal hard palate. This demonstrates the link between the maxilla and health issues.

The Palette itself starts to form about day 28-33 of gestation. By day 42-55 we have closure of the secondary palette. As the nose forms, the fusion of the medial nasal prominence with its contralateral counterpart creates the intermaxillary segment – which forms the primary palate (becomes the anterior 1/3 of the definitive palate). The intermaxillary segment also contributes to the labial component of the philtrum and the upper four incisors, think of it as the region that forms the nose, midline upper lip and the front 4 teeth region.

70 • SCOTT WUSTENBERG

A Early 6th week

B Early 6th week
- Medial nasal process
- Lateral nasal process
- Maxillary swelling
- Mandibular swelling

C Early 7th week

D Late 7th week
- Intermaxillary process

E 10th week
- Philtrum

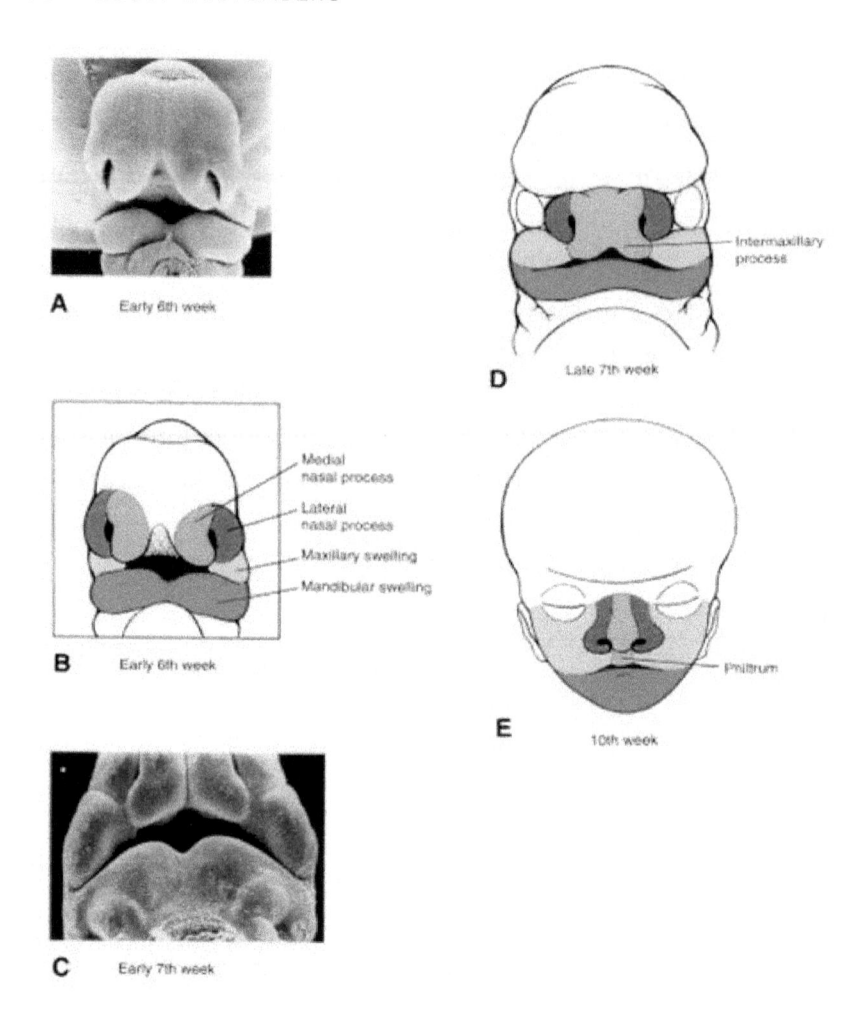

Image 8: Development of the face. *A, B,* In the sixth week, the nasal placodes of the frontonasal prominence invaginate to form the nasal pits and the lateral and medial nasal processes. *C, D,* In the seventh week, the medial nasal processes fuse at the midline to form the intermaxillary process. *E,* By the 10th week, the intermaxillary process forms the philtrum of the upper lip. (A, C, Photos courtesy of Dr. Arnold Tamarin.) http://www.columbia.edu/itc/hs/medical/humandev/2004/Chapt11-FacialPalatalDev.pdf

THE MAXILLARY PROMINENCES EXPAND MEDIALLY to give rise to the palatal shelves. These continue to advance medially, fusing superior to the tongue. Simultaneously, the developing mandible expands to increase the size of the oral cavity; this allows the tongue to drop out of the way of the growing palatal shelves. The palatal shelves then fuse with each other in the horizontal plane, and the nasal septum in the vertical plane, forming the secondary palate[lx].

This process is affected by the foetus swallowing during pregnancy, the palate needs the anterior and superior thrust of the tongue to develop, a firm pressure is required to mould the palette. Tethering of the tongue structure may alter this and lead to structural alteration. Please keep in mind that all this function is affected by alteration of cellular migration to the midline structure, DHFR alteration and apoptotic dysfunction as previously discussed.

This is very early on in the infant developmental process. Embryologically, the development of tongue is a very complicated process that starts around the fourth or fifth week of the gestation period, and its development has a marked influence on the oral cavity arising from the branchial arches.[lxi]

It continues to develop in a downwards pattern allowing separation from the floor of the mouth.

The anterior cranial base growth will progressively slow until ceasing about 7 years of age. While the true posterior portion of the cranial base continues growing till the child is in their late teens. This means that optimum intervention time to change the jaw and mandible growth structures is about 4 years until 7 years of age[lxii]. After that change is much harder as the mould is set. This flies in the face of traditional orthodontics which waits until adult dentition is between 11 and 15 years old before intervention.

Right time to intervene is not when you'd think

Of interest is the 1922 paper by Samuel Cohen MD Discussing Malocclusion and its far-reaching effect. He states that if the dental arch measures less than 28 mm by 4 years of age, it will not develop normally, without intervention. Dr Cohen was a strong advocate of early intervention and, suggested that mouth breathing, bottle feeding, and mushy food would have bad consequences for bite and facial development. Cohen further advocated for tonsil and adenoid removal to correct mouth breathing. In his paper he quotes a Dr Bogue. In his paper, Dr. Bogue states that "the child's brain at 6 years is within 40 grams of its weight at 19 years of age, suggesting that the most of the child's growing is done an d at 6 is very similar to adult in most regards; hence it is most important that all irregularities of the face and teeth should be corrected before the sixth year, while growth is at its maximum". He asserted that the growth of brain tissue is retarded mechanically by poor occlusion.

For these reasons and many others, the physician should be on the lookout for normal arches in children between the ages of 2 and 6 years[lxiii].

As you can see, what was known about 100 years ago appears to have been forgotten or hidden. From a breathing and brain function point of view, as a society we are missing the optimal window to change respiratory, sleep and neuro-emotional development by waiting until much later to make changes to the form, locking us in aberrant development patterns. Let alone the fact that therapy may not be based upon improving function as much as making teeth look pretty, locking teens into terrible trajectories that will create issues and symptoms such as apnoea and snoring in later life[lxiv]; which is associated with other health conditions which I will elucidate later.

Ankyloglossia and Craniofacial Developmental Dysfunction loops

Ankyloglossia and Craniofacial Developmental Dysfunction may contribute to abnormal patterns or behaviours leading to symptoms after birth. Obvious symptoms that can be seen include burping, positing, difficulty feeding, reflux, failure to thrive, a heightened startle response, poor sleep as well as disturbance of normal immune tolerance and ultimately disturbance to homeostasis. See the chart below[lxv]

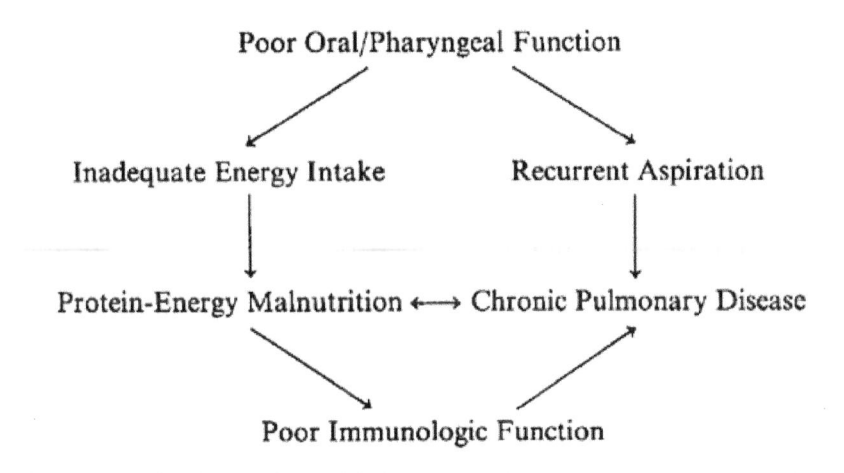

```
                    Poor Oral/Pharyngeal Function
                      /                    \
                     /                      \
          Inadequate Energy Intake      Recurrent Aspiration
                     |                         |
                     ↓                         ↓
          Protein-Energy Malnutrition ←→ Chronic Pulmonary Disease
                      \                      /
                       \                    /
                      Poor Immunologic Function
```

Diagram 2: Clinical sequelae of dysfunctional swallowing

If we consider the chart, we can appreciate that there are solid reasons that an infant may be sicklier, develop atopy[lxvi], asthma or reflux and be slow to make their milestones. According to The Royal Children's Hospital Melbourne[lxvii] reflux is common, affecting at least 40% of infants, which means that cranio-oral pharyngeal dysfunction or tongue fascial restriction may be a lot more common than we think, as is the consequences of it that create structural alteration potentiating airway consequences long term, such as hypopneas, anxiety, and apnoea.

What is Atopy?

Atopy is "a predisposition to an immune response against diverse antigens and allergens leading to CD4+, Th2 differentiation and overproduction of immunoglobulin E (IgE). The clinical consequence is an increased propensity to hypersensitivity or true allergic reactions"[lxviii].

Atopy has been demonstrated to be abundant in mouth breathing children with researchers suggesting that preventing mouth breathing may help prevent a series of issues, "In conclusion, this study demonstrated that mouth breathing is a risk factor for Allergic Dermatitis (AD) development, especially in children with a genetic family history of AD and can be a risk factor for tonsillitis (tonsillar hypertrophy) and class II dental malocclusion. Furthermore, mouth breathing during sleep (MBS) was closely related to allergic diseases and other respiratory diseases. Therefore, MBS is expected to be more harmful to children than MBD"[lxix]. From this we can see the basis of the doom loop forming.

Birth Trauma and interventional births

Traumatic, and abnormal births, including forceps suction, or C section births contribute to the alteration in structure and form leading to deviation in normal function and behaviour of the child's mouth and the wiring of the brain and the immune. The most extreme and obvious version is plagiocephaly. The infant's bones are not ossified, and the amount of force applied to the cranium to deliver the child can be enough to dislocate sutures, and start a pattern of cranial plate drift. It is considered sufficient to deliver the child at 14kg of suction force, which is well under the fracture stress point of 1000 Newtons or 102 kg of force suggested to fracture the Skull bone. However it is noted that it only takes 100g of force applied to the skull to induce a concussion, and that brain injury is a noted consequence of "The doctor uses forceps and birth-assistance tools with too much force on the infant's head"[lxx].

According to the Australian institute of Health and wellness[lxxi]: Over time, the proportion of women who had a vaginal non-instrumental birth has decreased, and the proportion of women who had a caesarean section birth has increased. Vaginal birth assisted by vacuum or forceps have remained relatively stable. In 2020 these statistics were:

- 50% of women had a non-instrumental vaginal birth (compared with 56% in 2010).
- 7.4% of women had a vaginal birth assisted by vacuum (compared with 8.1% in 2010).
- 5.2% of women had a vaginal birth assisted by forceps (compared with 4.0% in 2010).
- 37% of women had a caesarean section birth (compared with 32% in 2010)

There were 294,369 live births in Australia in 2020[lxxii]. (As an incidental point the birth rate is 1.7 per women indicating that Australia is still way below the magic 2.1 required to maintain the population at its current level, suggesting we are in decline). This indicates that approximately 147,184 children had an intervention and may have suffered trauma resulting in possible future craniofacial maldevelopment. We need to keep this in mind when assessing all paediatric patients. The stats are 1:2 and we note that developmental drift is commonly caused by mouth breathing resulting from any reason, including cranial trauma.

Craniofacial trauma is a noted cause of facial muscle tone issues and feeding issues post-partum. There is a huge amount of force applied to the baby's head during delivery even if considered largely normal.

From Linda Smiths 2007 paper on the impact of birth practices on the breastfeeding dyad we find that the labour and birth, subjects the infant's skull to mechanical forces that may disrupt bony structure, as well as affect cranial and thoracic nerves, while also compressing the brain and central nervous system structures. Keeping in mind this is the supposed normal force.

Her work is considered seminal that it studies the 12 paired cranial nerves that issue from the brain and, like spinal nerves, have both afferent (sensory) fibres and efferent (motor) fibres.

Six of the 12 cranial nerves that are involved in sucking, swallowing, and/or breathing, pass through tiny foramens between the bony segments of the cranium. Mechanical forces to the cranium during labour can disrupt nerve function or cause nerve entrapment. Forces from excess or unusual pressures can potentially disrupt nerve function for a longer time[lxxiii] or lead to permanent functional impairment.

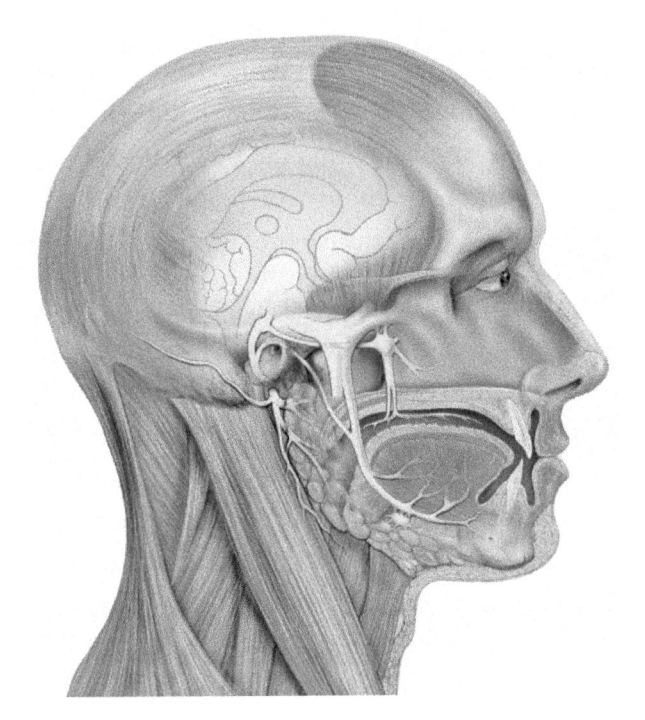

Image 9: This image illustrates the Deep Facial Cranial nerve and Trigemnal nerve which supply the tongue, and areas of the TMJ and superficial parts of the ear. https://commons.wikimedia.org/wiki/File: Head_deep_facial_trigeminal.png Patrick J. Lynch, medical illustrator, CC BY 2.5 https:// creativecommons.org/licenses/by/2.5, via Wikimedia Commons

Forceps and vacuum use can directly or indirectly affect breastfeeding. No studies yet report on direct effects of instruments on breastfeeding. However, lactation professionals frequently deal with indirect results. Hall et al[lxxiv]. investigated factors predicting breast feeding cessation and found that vacuum vaginal delivery was a strong predictor of early cessation. Computerised tomography (CT) scans of symptomatic term infants observed that poor or disturbed feeding is one sign of intracranial bleeding. Vacuum extraction devices contribute to increased rates of hyperbilirubinemia and kernicterus secondary to the creation of cephalohematomas and/or bruising. Jaundiced babies are more lethargic and therefore feed poorly; conversely, poor feeding can cause or exacerbate jaundice. Jaundice is a frequent reason for supplementing the breast- fed baby; therefore, any practices that increase the risk of jaundice will nearly always have a negative effect on exclusive breastfeeding.

Forceps use can cause bruising and nerve damage to the sides of the infant cranium, causing the jaw to deviate to the paralysed side when the mouth is open. This is likely to end up in a long-term deviation to open mouth breathing changes in facial structure which are all strongly associated with sleep airway disturbances such as UARS, which is a precursor to apnoea. The bruising can cause swelling and inflammation in the jaw joint, altering the normal action and increasing feeding discomfort for the dyad pair.

6

Neurological Development patterns

CNS development is a bottom, midline up and out occurrence. It starts at the lower brain stem, spinal cord and cerebellum via primitive reflexes and feedback loops. Phase 2 of development is in the midbrain (visual and auditory localization region) limbic areas allowing for secure attachment and the ability to localize self in space, this also starts our ability to derive a threat and the speed of which it is coming at us, along with determining left and right. These behaviours are driven by primitive reflexes and the more mature postural reflexes. Casar described the Asymmetric Tonic neck Reflex as a privileged position that allows the infant to focus on its surrounding and orientate its eyes to the hand mouth pair. By the second month post-partum vision is associated with shaping whole body posture control. Postural structure is dependent entirely on spatial associating of objects[lxxv]. By 3 months the infants' arms do not participate in visual tracking, this is the transition from the ATNR to postural reflex control of the head and trunk.

The third phase of CNS development as we go up is cortical development. This begins in the cross over phase of primitive reflexes becoming postural versions and learning to initiate motor movement patterns by choice. As the pathways are laid down, we develop higher thinking which lead to language and learning and action, first beginning with survival behaviours then in all goes well heading into the abstract.

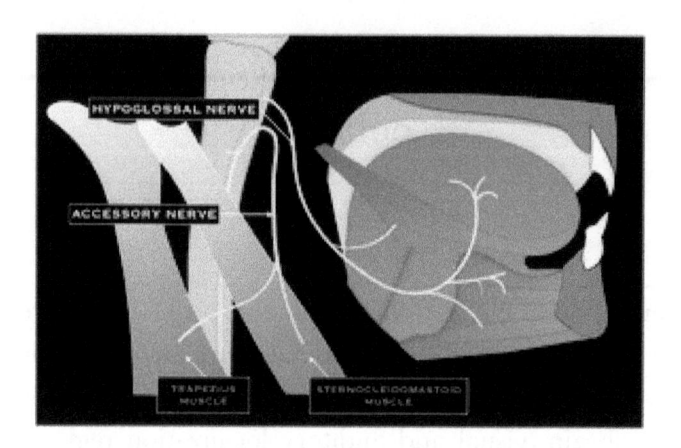

Image 10: Schematic drawing of the accessory and hypoglossal nerves, which supply the tongue, trapezius muscle and sternocleidomastoid muscle. Romano, N., Federici, M. & Castaldi, A. Schematic drawing of the accessory and hypoglossal nerves.png

The neurological control of the tongue is located in the brainstem and encompasses postural and autonomic reflexes which have been developing starting at 4 months of gestation as well as conscious muscular control, it is tied heavily into the vagus nerve and is connected to our limbic system. In fact, it is intrinsic to the soothing capacity and if dysregulated may set the person up for maladaptive stress and anxiety responses as an adult.

An important point to keep in mind is that Babies will feel pain as a nociceptive response, a noxious stimuli which drives a stress and startle response, however they cannot verbalise this as pain, but only in a manner that mirrors all stress responses such as crying and upset, which can facilitate windup loops and learned stress adaptive response, including avoiding sticking things in its mouth. This is important to keep in mind post any intervention surgery for ankyloglossia, as stretching the tongue directly while a wound is open soon after surgery may not be in the child interest as against touching gently in a playful fashion, stroking as well as feeding to facilitate normal function.

Move the tongue as consciously as possible, with as minimal intervention as possible. Encourage elevation, especially of the posterior tongue.

Nerve innervation of the mouth and Tongue

MOTOR INNERVATION

Motor output = Glossopharyngeal, spinal accessory and the vagus nerve. Most motor action of the tongue is supplied by the hypoglossal nerve (CN XII), both intrinsic and most extrinsic muscles *except* the **palatoglossus**, which is supplied by the vagus (CV X). Motor innervation gives ability to move muscles. This is efferent nerves which carries information out from the Central Nervous System (CNS).

Position sense of the tongue is limited as it has no muscle spindles, thus spatial position regulation is conditioned by the borders of the mouth the teeth, hard palette and cheek mucosal membranes, neural dysregulation of structures such as the TMJ (especially in cat 2 situations) may lead to a greater likelihood of biting the tongue. That said all spatial muscle patterns of movement and feedback is learned by the baby over time due to use.

SENSORY SUPPLY

The sensory component of the tongue is divided into the anterior 2/3 and posterior 1/3. These areas are supplied by different nerves.

There are two main class of sensory input: **general** (touch, temperature, and pressure) and **special** sensation (taste). These are afferent nerves carrying information to the CNS.

> **Anterior 2/3 General:** supplied by the trigeminal nerve (CN V), which has three branches: ophthalmic (CN V1), maxillary (CN V2) and mandibular (CN V3). Out of those three branches, the mandibular (CN V3) branch gives rise to another smaller branch called the lingual nerve, which supplies the anterior 2/3 of the tongue (and that is general sensation).
> **Anterior 2/3 Special:** This is supplied by the facial nerve (CN VII) from a branch called the chorda tympani. The chorda tympani *hitchhike* onto the lingual nerve to get to the oral cavity. Hitchhiking nerves means they share a common path.

During surgeries as seen in the *Journal of Anatomy* paper **'Surgical anatomy and pathology of the middle ear'** damage to the chorda tympani can occur and patients may lose the sensation of taste to a certain degree[lxxvi].

> "During any middle ear surgery, the surgeon is confronted with the course of the chorda tympani. Sometimes, especially in the endaural approach towards the stapes in otosclerosis surgery, the chorda tympani has to be stretched and moved aside to gain better access to the middle ear and especially to the ossicular chain. Although the chorda is flexible and hence

moving it temporarily aside is possible, this stretching may result in taste disturbances. Fortunately, these tend to disappear after a short time, as the sense of taste is transmitted by a total of six nerves on both sides of the mouth (nerve VII, IX, X), which after a while recoup the full sense. Still, the chorda may be accidentally injured, for example when removing parts of the bony ear canal in the dorsal aspect, or by accidently drying up of the nerve fibres due to the heat generated from the hot light of the surgical microscope or simply by contacting the bare nerve due to mechanical action.

Posterior 1/3 General and Special: both are supplied by the glossopharyngeal nerve (CV IX).

From a practical purpose clinically, we use 7 out of about 200 oral reflexes to determine function in an infant, we also use taste in an older individual. Taste function can be implied by putting a drop of sugar on the tongue of the newborn and looking at sucking rate, if it increases it suggests chemoception (thus taste) of sweet is active and processing in the brain creating a motor output increase.

Glossopharyngeal nerve carries sensory information, as well as parasympathetic fibres and the efferent motor output. It provides taste as well as saliva production and is essential to elevate the larynx and pharynx in swallowing and during speaking, it also has a communicating branch to the vagus it also supplies a portion of the tympanic membrane. This could have a link with tongue issues and ear pain.

The vagus nerve is a major part of the control and regulation of the autonomic nervous system (ANS) and contributes significantly to social and emotional function. It innervates most of our organs and provides feedback loops to most of our emotional hyper thinking for example a gut feeling.

Vagal tone is associated with nourishment and general good health. In infants' low tone is associated with poor growth and weight gain. The vagus nerve and ANS function is associated with rest digest versus fight flight, thus if the child develops wind up loops due to swallowing issues from tongue tie, or post-surgery pain, the tonal balance may shift leading to digestive irritability, heart and respiratory rate increase which leads to pH imbalance in the bloodstream.

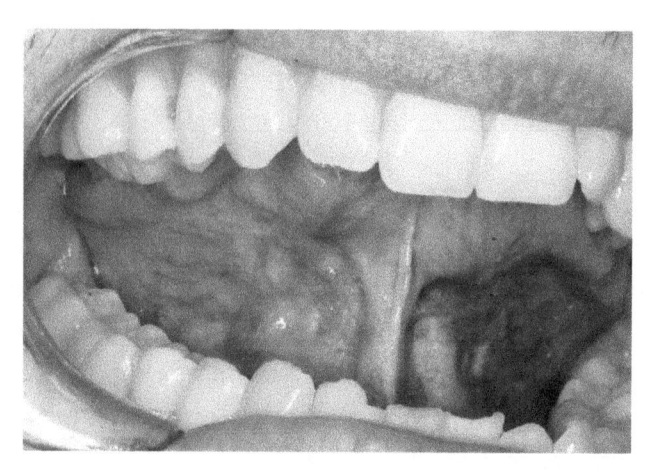

Image 11: Demonstrate the tongue and lingual frenulum before a lingual frenulum reduction surgery.

First Principles • 85

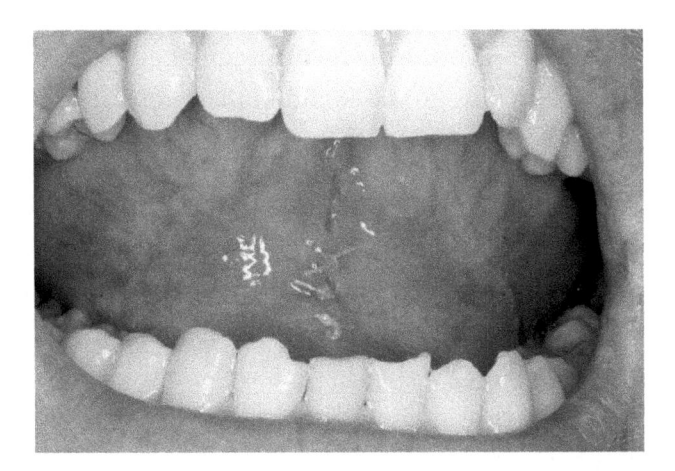

Images 12: The above image show the same Tongue after of a lingual frenulum reduction surgery.

A PAPER by Tiffany Field et al suggests that Low baseline vagus tone is noted in prenatally depressed mother and infants as well as in autistic kids and suggests that's it is a marker for infant risk conditions. Whereas vagal toning activity such as massage, touch, skin contact, face to face interaction improved growth and development. Further it is noted, that high facial expressively is associated with better vagal tone in children, from which we can extrapolate that oral facial restrictions that alter structure of the face and muscle use may alter vagal tone and ANS function. Therefore, any of the previous mention issues, tongue tie, mouth breathing, structural cartilaginous alteration, birth trauma, poor vagal tone etc, might have far reaching and unintended consequences, even after correction of facial structural issues.

The trigeminal nerve provides huge amount of sensory feedback to the brain. The motor branch is to the muscles of mastication. The Trigeminal nerve will become overactivated if swallowing movements become dysregulated, this overstimulation in a feeding pair can cause chomping on the nipple. If the trigeminal nerve over fires it will turn down the vagus nerve response this may lead to ANS reflexes to be situation inappropriate

The major nuclei involved include the Nucleus Tractus solitarius (NTS) and the Intermediate Nucleus of the Medulla (InM), and the hypoglossal nucleus, these co-ordinate the head neck input, spatial awareness of tongue jaw and teeth and the motor patterns of the tongue and upper airway, to allow the ANS to develop appropriate firing patterns thus if we have oral dysfunction it can lead to airway dysregulation, and over use of head/neck muscles to compensate for appropriate action.

Sympathetic Dominance - Long Term issues

Arguably all children are born sympathetically dominant in a heightened state of stress/tone, the point of the mother child dyad bonding is for the child to use latch, feeding connection, skin contact sound and the mother's cortex to learn to soothe and regulate the nervous system, we are built for survival and learn to be calm. If there are issues of the oral structures that cause dysregulated feedback loops, (nociception /poor latch, aerophagy/reflux etc) a lack of connection to mum especially due to changed feeding style, (bottle vs breast) we may struggle to activate the appropriate reflexes in the CNS, this may cause compensation in the nervous system, increased wiring to vigilance (sensitivity to catecholamines) poorer HRV and poorer growth outcomes.

The tongue is strongly connected to midline systems including the vermis of the cerebellum. If there is poor tongue function early in life this can show as low tone in the midline structures, and express as weakness in those muscles, this includes the hip girdle, shoulder girdle, lips, eyes, and neck. Dysregulation of which can lead to further developmental delay and long-term issues.

The cerebellum is involved in all motor activity and learning, this is super important as the Cerebellum is strongly involved in emotional learning. All thoughts are motor patterns thus emotions which are thoughts, always have a motor pathway involved. Thus, if there is an issue with the first motor sensory tool the baby uses (the Tongue and Mouth structures, then eyes), we may find issues with all higher functional/emotional learning.

This gives a greater emphasis to the concept of breast is best.

The 4 phases of swallowing

It's essential to understand how we swallow, as dysregulation of these actions creates compensatory actions which alters structural growth. Below is an outline of what normal action occurs in the neonate and in the adult.

1. Oral preparatory phase = sucking and mastication, either the breast/bottle or a bolus of food enters the anterior mouth and is prepped for swallowing by the tongue, cheeks and teeth either sucking or chewing depending on age of the person.
2. Oral transitory phase = when the tongue moves the breast or bolus to the back of the. Mouth/pharynx with a progressive contractile motion, think of a Mexican wave type motion.
3. Pharyngeal phase = where the tongue elevates to the hard palate closing the nasopharynx, the vocal cords are closed by movement of the hyoid bone in an anterior, superior motion which tips the epiglottis inferior, the

muscles of the pharynx also contract to move the bolus towards the oesophagus.
4. Oesophageal phase = is when the tongue, epiglottis and the hyoid return to their resting position, the bolus moves into the oesophagus and the soft palette drops inferior allowing the laryngeal fold to reopen.

Deviation of this process can lead to swallowing issues, such as aerophagy, refluxing, particulate matter ending up in the lungs or choking.

Under-function of the vagus control for any reason can cause the nasopharynx to not close properly leading to choking - this can also cause lipstick shaped nipples, in the feeding Mother. Therefore, if you note this sign in yourself or your patients, then the child should be assessed for a tongue tie or swallowing disorder.

Hypertension in the hyoid muscles will occur if the tongue cannot elevate properly, such as due to a tie, or weakness /paralysis of the Palatoglossus.

During the suck swallow breathe reflex in a baby, the breath should always be nasal, and should continue as the bolus of milk moves from the nipple to the oropharynx (posterior of mouth)

As the bolus enters the vestibule of the pharynx, an initial puff of expiration breath precedes breath holding which protects the airway, the Larynx is then closed and the milk bolus (or food) moves past the larynx, down the throat. As it passes below the larynx, the breath is fully expelled, and the cycle starts again.

Adult versus Infant Swallowing

There is a big innervation difference between adult and infant swallowing. Infants can breathe and swallow at the same time, adults can't achieve this. This presents an issue for a baby with neural dysregulation, or structure issues leading to motor issues. If the rhythm fails, fluid can end in the wrong hole and aspiration, or other serious consequence may ensue.

It's noted that occlusion and posture of the tongue in the mouth plays a key role in the development of acquired postural reflexes, A study by Lumbau demonstrated that swallowing is able to modulate postural control, and they further went on to say that if the postural syndrome is not properly intercepted and dealt with in the infant it may turn into an irreversible Musculo skeletal disorder, in the adult.

Postural change experiments in rats are shown to alter spine development by changing jaw occlusion. Think of this in a scenario of mouth breathing, this may lead to bony alteration in the spinal structure and how we ambulate.

There is also a large link between eye function and control of the eye muscles with muscle and osseous development from oral function. This occurs for many reasons, think about the high arch palette altering the sinus airway affecting the bones floor of the eye socket, let alone the neurological cross talk of neuronal pools that need to either recruit support to make an essential action occur such as swallowing, this occurs in the homologous columns, or perhaps that the inhibition of one neuronal area fails and leaks symptoms due to fatigue, or an excess excitation to make another area work . Considering that the eyes and the tongue are both midline structures with brain stem pools above one another in the homologous column and a vermal cerebellar output, crosstalk becomes highly likely especially in a poorly myelinated system as one finds in an infant.

As a practical example, if the jaw/TMJ is dysfunctional perhaps due to narrowness of the sphenoidal plate, and being used in a compensatory fashion we might see an increase in Trigeminal hyperexcitability cross linking to the oculomotor muscles. This may lead to poor eye stability and vertiginous type symptoms, further we know that improved saccades help postural stability, and the reverse is capably true.

Nasal breathing

There is a strong functional preference towards nasal breathing, with the airways having several jobs that they are meant to do, including:

- filtering air with cilia
- Filtering with nasal mucosa
- Humidifying
- Heating
- The release of nitric oxide as an antibiotic into the airflow from the sinuses
- Adenoids and then tonsils cleaning the air.

If the mouth is open to breath all the cleaning is done by the tonsils in the pharynx. This is not ideal and is especially worsened by the child sleeping or breathing in an environment with increased toxic loads such as mould spores, dust, dust mites, bacteria, or other particulates.

As we previously mentioned, irritated sinuses can lead to the Doom Loop, which leads to greater difficulty in nasal breathing especially during sleep as enlargement of the tonsils can occlude the airway both from nasal and mouth breathing and contributes to snoring and apnoea. The lips and cheek muscles act as one part of the jelly mould, the tongue thrust up and forward in a normally developing child will lead to optimal maxilla and jaw development, this is a dome shaped arch, like that in the Sistine chapel. If the tongue sits down and forward in the oral space the bone development is not adequately pressurised or splayed and results in suboptimal bone development and short rami causing teeth to become crowded in the jaws. This creates a maxilla that has a gothic chapel roof, narrow and tall, which impacts on the nasal air space, leading to septal dilation, especially after orthodontic involvement.

The four elements of good posture of the tongue and mouth

1. Tongue lightly suctioned to the roof of the mouth.
2. Lips gently sealed without strain.
3. Nasal breathing
4. No activity of the muscles around the mouth during subconscious swallowing

Good oral posture is encouraged by discouraging habits such as the use of pacifiers, or finger/thumb sucking, along with prolonged sippy cup use. There are no sippy cups in nature, that's not how we learned to use our mouths to drink for previous millennia. These all alter lip seal and how the muscles of the mouth move, often leaving the lips apart and greater capacity for bacteria to enter the oral cavity and leading to infection of teeth, dental carries, and tonsil issues.

Any time the muscles of the face or mouth do not work correctly we call this a myofunctional disorder which includes during suction, swallowing, breathing chewing or speech, regardless of age of patient. However, from a developmental point of view form follows function, thus before you see the crooked, crowded teeth, a high arch, or large tonsils, we should be able to see the warning signs which herald later issues.

Myofunctional disorders tend to be glossed over and not be given as much significance as they should. They don't have a true screening program, and only get collected as an afterthought when a problem has developed. We seem to take it for granted that development is perfect and that issues such as crowded teeth are just structural things, and not that they are driven from myofunctional discrepancy.

From the book Sleep Breath thrive, myofunctional disorders include:

- Open mouth breathing
- Infant latching or sucking problems.
- Poor swallowing and excessive air intake while feeding
- Reflux like symptoms in infancy
- Tongue/lip/buccal ties
- Use of pacifiers/finger/thumb sucking
- Overuse of pouch foods bottles and or snippy cups.
- Nasal obstruction enlarged tonsils and adenoids.
- Allergies and nasal congestion
- Poor swallowing and estuation tube clearance - recurrent ear infection or glue ear
- Soft overly processed diets which require little chewing
- Chewing and swallowing difficulties
- Messy open mouth chewing
- Drooling
- Snoring
- Teeth grinding clenching and bruxism.

- Lisps, speech articulations issues, particularly with n, l, a, d, s and z
- Nail biting
- Chewing on clothes hair or objects
- Other consequences of oral myofunctional disorder can be seen with picky eating or a preference for soft food.
- The tongue thrusting between the teeth to help form.
- Choking during mealtimes
- The need for liquid during meals to help the swallow.
- Excess and inappropriate placement of tension on the lips.

The above list includes many symptoms patterns that modern children display and are brushed off as quite normal. Parents are often told as I was that there is nothing to be concerned about, that your child will grow out of it. My observation is children don't grow out of structural or functional issues without intervention and rehabilitation, they compensate. Either effectively or poorly. If the compensation pattern is poor then it is more likely to show up sooner, and if the parents are affluent enough then an intervention will be started. However, most interventions are to treat the consequences of the myofunctional problem, not necessarily the cause. For example, the child may be taken to a paediatric gastroenterologist, and be given a proton pump inhibitor, they may see a speech language therapist to help facial tone and word pronunciation, or they may have orthodontic work performed at 12 years old to improve the bite. All of these interventions are useful, as part of the symptom continuum, but none addressed the oral fascial restriction, nor looked at nasal versus mouth breathing, and none considered the consequences to sleep.

If the tongue remains tethered, if swallow is not correct and functional, if nasal breathing patency is not established and appropriate sleep is not generated then the continuum will progress, and further symptom patterns will evolve.

Consequences of mouth breathing

Nasal breathing is a pillar of health generally and without it, disease progression is a slow grind onwards. The obvious signs of which will be seen with dry mouth in the patient, along with chapped lips from the air going across them all the time, bad breath, inflamed gums, and gingivitis are all part of it, as well as increase dental decay and plaque, acidification of the mouth, all due to the decline in the saliva production as the mouth is dry.

Further signs include increased tension in the neck, scalp, and facial muscles, especially around the jaw. Mouth breathers are more likely to suffer migraines and tension headaches, this can be due to low oxygen in circulation, blood acidification and its poor oxygen release to the tissues and electrolyte imbalance (think calcium and magnesium to start) as well as from over activation of muscle spindles leading to trigger points and pain syndromes.

Think about this from a recruitment point of view, if you're having difficulty breathing due to airway occlusion the brain recruits more muscles to cause inhalation and increases tension in them until airflow is achieved or until you wake up (if asleep), this also can occur during wake times, especially due to poorly learned breathing habits.

The neck derived headaches are termed cervicogenic headaches and are common is **UARS** (upper airway resistance syndrome) sufferers. The upper airway resistance syndrome (UARS) is a recently described form of sleep-disordered breathing in which repetitive increases in resistance to airflow within the upper airway led to brief arousals and daytime somnolence[lxxvii].

These patients will commonly attend the Chiropractor, Physio, Osteopath, or massage therapist on a regular basis to seek relief from the "My neck and shoulders are always tight" complaint. Sadly, the therapy does not last long, and the tension rebuilds, due to the issue occurring as a defence mechanism to protect the airway while asleep.

In the child increased risk of upper airway problems including rhinitis, sinusitis, and ear infections. This commonly is linked to increased use of antibiotics along with enlarged tonsils and adenoids and is an independent factor in the aetiology of asthma. Therefore, we can see that if you're not breathing through your nose well as a child there are many seemingly unrelated symptom patterns you can develop in your adult life, not commonly associated with maldevelopment of breathing. Headaches and migraines are commonly treated either as a pain syndrome with drugs, a MSK issue with adjustment at the Chiropractor or in extreme cases surgical intervention to ablate nerves.

Tongue Posture and the CNS

By this stage I hope to have you realise that tongue posture is an essential element of craniofacial development and is integrated into CNS development very early in the piece. Tongue posture is altered by mouth breathing and tongue posture can lead to mouth breathing especially during REM phases of sleep when the muscle paralysis occurs, and muscle tone lowers in the sleep cycle.

Alteration of tongue/oral posture and poor tone in the muscles contributes to apnoea and hypopnea events driving lower oxygen saturation and increased carbon dioxide in the blood stream. The alteration in CO2 upwards, creatures a shift in the acid base balance of the blood leading to acidification, and potential stress on the pancreas where bicarbonate is made and released to keep pH in all body compartments in range. This could also have implications for bone development and calcification of the structure, especially in mouth breathing infants.

Cranial Developmental Drift

Open mouth breathing for any reason is associated with a phenomenon called cranial developmental drift. The children's face slowly deviates away from normal growth. Leading to an adult with structural postural change including a long face, narrow through the jaw and maxilla, this is also called an adenoid face. Seen with more prominent protruding teeth, and an incapacity to keep the lips sealed, recursion of the mandible, and slackening off the jaw and jaw muscles, the teeth will then tend to become crowded and crooked in the arch. The narrow palette with the high arch is an airway risk factor which is associated with disturbed sleep and breathing (OSA) leading to consequences in adulthood we will discuss further later.

Mouth breathing is associated with an increase in airway resistance termed upper airway resistance syndrome (UARS) by 2.5 times. The consequence is airway collapsibility, snoring and OSA and or hypopnea, which gives reduced restive sleep.

As a side note to clue us all into impact chronic Hypopneas are noted to increase dementia risk, so should not be viewed as less dangerous that full OSA.

It is not surprising that sleep is not restorative in this scenario, as the airway must be defended by the brain at all costs, and the brain will release catecholamines (cortisol and adrenaline) to tighten the airway, and partially raise the body out of the sleep state to a greater level of consciousness and alertness without full consciousness of this happening. This is termed sleep fragmentation. It is one of the most innocuous and most dangerous conditions that humans suffer. It leads to all and any disease you can think of.

I know that sounds like a bold statement, but it is true.

The emotional dysregulation makes a lot of sense given that the brain is a pattern and sense generator trying to make sense of the world. If it senses the bloodstream/body is filled with stress/threat hormones then it runs the threat program, sadly if you cannot find the cause of the threat, as the monster is not in the room (it's your tongue/airway choking you in your sleep when you did not see it with your conscious brain) it will leave you uneasy and constantly looking for the monster, this resembles vigilance and anxiety.

Fragmentation of sleep is associated with many long-term consequences, including increased interleukin 6 (IL6) production, increased blood sugar, insulin resistance, weight gain, hormonal dysregulation, and social emotional problems including depression and anxiety.

IL-6 is our immediate early response to organism threat and is promptly and transiently produced in response to infections and tissue injuries, and adrenal chemical response, it contributes to host defence through the stimulation of acute phase responses, haematopoiesis, and immune reactions[lxxviii].

Further to this we know that chronic high amounts of IL6 release is shown to damage the serotonergic receptors and increase pain sensitization, as well as other aspects of neurocognition and mood. Serotonin and the serotonin receptors modulate anxiety along with dopamine and other inhibitory neurotransmitters and our capacity to sleep as part of the melatonin production cycle, in fact pain sensitisation and inflammation will stop the person sleeping and induce a scenario more likely to fragment sleep.

Signs of sleep apnoea in children

While not as commonly considered children also suffer OSA and hypopneas, not just adults, the following list are signs to watch for. Keep in mind unless they have a cold the child should never sleep with their mouths open.

1. Snoring: Children with sleep apnoea may snore loudly and frequently during sleep.
2. Breathing pauses: Children with sleep apnoea may have periods of time during sleep where they stop breathing or have shallow breathing.
3. Restless sleep: Children with sleep apnoea may have trouble sleeping through the night and may be restless or thrash around in bed.
4. Daytime sleepiness: Children with sleep apnoea may be excessively tired or have difficulty staying awake during the day.
5. Bedwetting: Children with sleep apnoea may experience bedwetting due to the disrupted sleep caused by the condition.

Issues From the Tonsils and Adenoids

I want to take an aside to discuss a factor involved in airway issues, this being the tonsils and adenoids. The tonsils are a group of lymphoid organs that are part of the immune system. They are located in the aerodigestive tract, also known as Waldeyer's tonsillar ring, and consist of the adenoid tonsil, two tubal tonsils, two palatine tonsils, and the lingual tonsils. These organs help to fight infections by producing tonsil tissue.

In young children, the tonsils become larger and then should shrink to adult size by the age of 8 to 12 years. The adenoids are a patch of lymphoid tissue that is located at the back of the nasal airway. Like the tonsils, they help to fight infections and clean the air that flows into the lungs by trapping harmful bacteria and viruses.

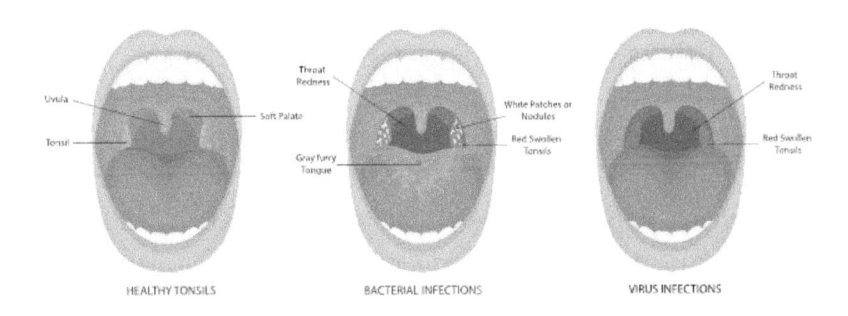

Image 13: Demonstrating stages of the Tonsils, normal, bacterial infection, Viral infection. Courtesy of istock images

The adenoids are located in the nasal airway, where the back of the nose meets the throat. They cannot be seen through the mouth without special instruments. Adenoids also become larger in young children and shrink to adult size by the age of 8 to 12 years.

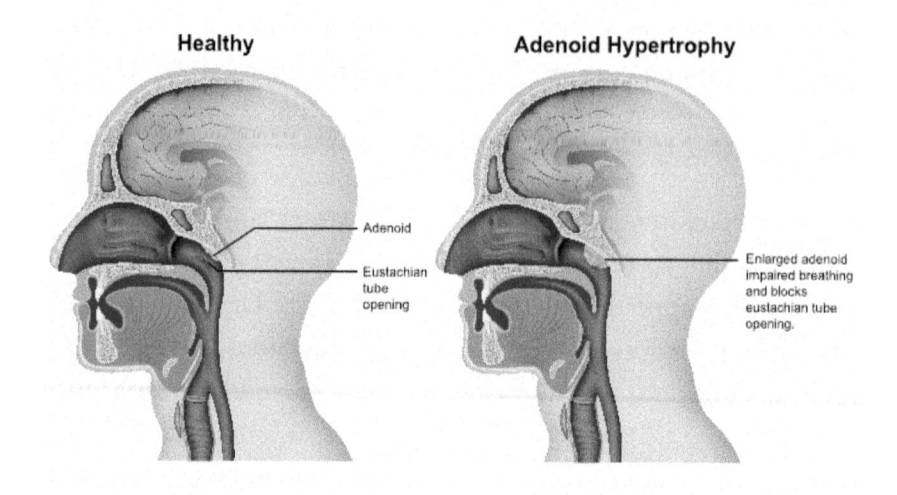

Image 14: Demonstrate Healthy and enlarged Adenoid tissue in the upper airway. Note the encroachment into the airway which will impede airflow, and lead to issues such as mouth breathing, UARS, and further infection. Courtesy of iStock images

According to Kim et al[lxxix] "Adeno-tonsillar hypertrophy is the major pathophysiological mechanism underlying obstructive sleep apnoea (OSA) and recurrent tonsillitis (RI) in children". Their work found that enhanced local and systemic inflammation in children with OSA promotes tonsillar proliferation. They found that proinflammatory cytokines, such as TNF-α, IL-6, and IL-1α, were highly expressed in OSA-derived tonsils. This raises an interesting counterpoint as to causation. We know in some cases that the enlargement of tonsils and adenoids are a cause of OSA, especially the hypertrophy of lingual tonsils after adenotonsillectomy[lxxx], causing the airway to be encroached upon, leading to snoring, open mouth breathing and upregulation of the aforementioned inflammatory response.

ADENOIDS

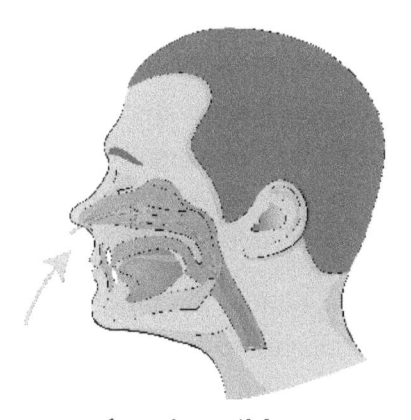

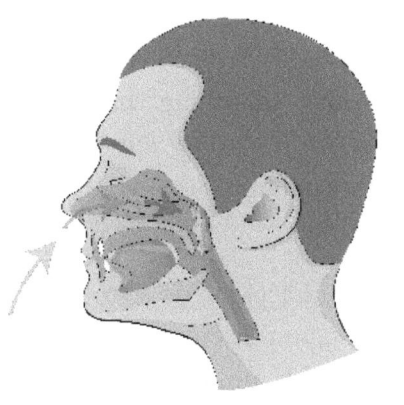

free breathing

respiratory failure in adenoids

Image 15: Demonstrates easy airflow versus respiratory failure with enlarged adenoids. Courtesy of iStock images.

Note the obstruction of the nasal airflow in the upper airway created by the enlarged adenoids. This occurs during daytime breathing but is often worse when lying supine at night, due to the mechanics of the airspace. The end result is a reduction in clear air intake, obstruction of the upper airway, an increase in upper airway resistance, opening of the mouth to breath, an increase in intake of environmental toxins to the airway and tonsils, increasing further likelihood of breathing difficulty and an increased possibility of hypopnea developing, which in the long term if unresolved may become OSA, but is noted to be causative of blood flow restriction to the brain, an increase in blood pressure, stroke and CVD risk and many other diseases.

However, as we have discussed, open mouth breathing leads to airway inflammation and upregulation of the immune system, both in the throat, the lungs, and then systematically as a consequence. The T cells are highly proliferative in the tonsils of children and are associated with increased production of proinflammatory cytokines which leads to the tonsils becoming enlarged. My point about this inflammatory loop either way, is that both scenarios, whether due to tonsilitis or due to open mouth breathing have increased inflammation, dysfunction mouth breathing and potentially lead to developmental drift in the midline cranial structures, which we have mentioned previously and will go into more detail about soon.

A tonsillectomy is a surgical procedure to remove the tonsils. An adenotonsillectomy is a surgical procedure to remove both the adenoids and tonsils. I had both tissues removed at about 5 years of age, after repeated bouts of ear nose and throat infections, and being diagnosed with glue ear.

Enlarged tonsils or adenoids can cause snoring in children, UARS, and obstructive Sleep apnoea. This is not normal and can have negative effects on sleep quality, behaviour, learning and osseous facial development. If a child is snoring, experiencing restlessness during sleep, or experiencing pauses in breathing (apnoea), surgery may be recommended. They may also be very hot-headed during sleep and quite sweaty. The beginning of hot Flashes but not menopause clearly. It's actually likely to be due to vagal dysregulation and upregulation of adrenal hormones as part of the protective compensations to protect the airway. It can also be partially due to chronic low-grade infection in the upper airway; however this sign continues in children that are not noted to be infectious.

Tonsillitis, or inflammation of the tonsils, can also warrant surgery independent of the airway consequences. If a child is experiencing frequent and severe tonsillitis that is affecting their schooling or daily life, or if they have long-lasting tonsillitis that does not respond well to antibiotic treatment, a tonsillectomy or adenotonsillectomy may be recommended. As a general guideline, this may be considered if a child has:

- 6 or more infections in 1 year
- 4 to 5 infections each year for the past 2 years
- 3 infections each year for the past 3 years

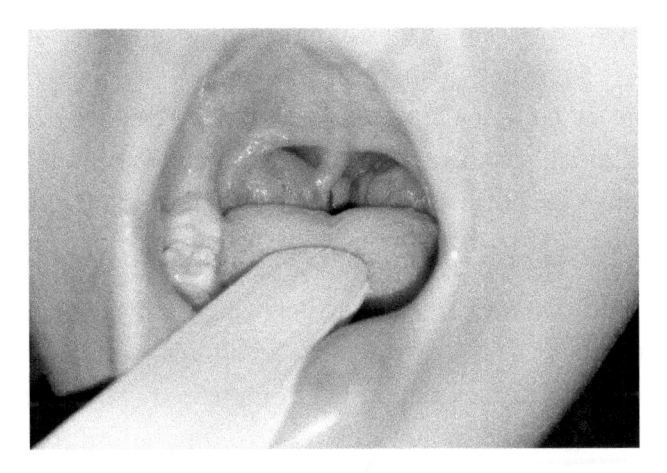

Image 16: Demonstrates infected tonsils. Look at the narrowing of posterior oral space, this will affect the nasal airway as well as the airflow from mouth breathing, notwithstanding the ability to swallow food due to the encroachment of the lymph tissue into posterior mouth, pharynx, and airway. From istock images.

The success rate for a tonsillectomy or adenotonsillectomy for improving or curing symptoms of sleep-disordered breathing is between 80% and 97%. The procedure is more likely to be successful if there are no other underlying conditions, such as obesity, contributing to the sleep-disordered breathing. In rare cases, the adenoids may grow back after surgery[lxxxi].

UARS halts normal Facial and Cranial growth

Increased nasal resistance has a dramatic effect on the maxillomandibular skeleton, halting growth[lxxxii] and bringing about adaptive changes in the soft tissues that are associated with deviation in jaw posture[lxxxiii] and tongue activity[lxxxiv].

Obstruction of nasal airflow equivalent to that occurring in UARS is known to induce functional changes in the nasomaxillary complex and on the mandible. Studies performed on newborn rhesus monkeys, created developmental consequences for bony structure of their faces, and airway.

The maxilla development was restricted as was the nose and upper jaw in size and shape. Further when displacement of the mandible occurred, it led to mouth breathing. Mouth breathing that developed in association with increased nasal resistance (UARS), caused the infant monkey to be mouth open and breathing through the mouth, both when awake and asleep.

The interesting thing is that these changes which led to the narrowing of the cranial skeleton, palette, and face, were shown to be reversible if the experimental nasal airway resistance was withdrawn while the infant monkey was still in its developmental phase[lxxxv]. This indicates that if we intervene early enough in human subjects a lot of the damage should be reversible avoiding much of the long-term consequences and hopefully a decline in progression down the continuum.

The issue seems to be that we do not appear to be diagnosing tongue tie and airway problems, early enough if at all. Orthodontic application is generally performed at 12-15 years of age which is very late from a cranial bone development viewpoint. In normal individuals, 60% of facial growth is attained by 6 years and about 90% by 11–12 years of age, thus by

15 years, the skeleton is patently ancient adult, and only 10% growth is expected in the facial structure and much of the abnormality is set for life.

In the monkey infants soft-tissue changes were seen, such as development of a triangular upper lip (think a pert sweetheart lip with breathy open mouth seen in all the starlets in Hollywood) and a groove within the tongue, preceding the skeletal and dental adaptation and were evident within the first 6 months of nasal obstruction.

This demonstrates the significant impact that nasal breathing has on development of normal bone structure and that mouth breathing for any reason leads development down the wrong path. The genioglossus, geniohyoid, inferior orbicularis oris, and lip-elevator fibres were behaviourally recruited, seemly to enhance breathing survival when the normal pathway was not available to the child. Miller found that the neuromuscular changes extend beyond the period of obstruction which will continue to effect structural development, leading to the classic open bite, or cross bite structural positions which we see in children with poor nasal breathing.

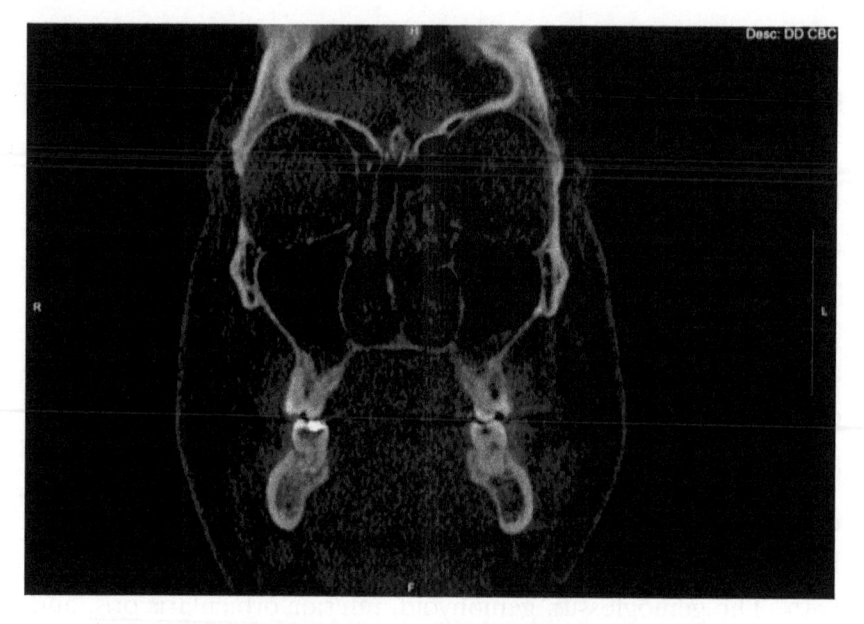

Image 17: This image shows the nasal airway, and the orbits and bite. Note the deviation of the septum away to the right of midline, the thickening of the turbinates and increased nasal mucosa, with limitation of airflow through the nose contributing to UARS.

Other Sleep Consequences of the Continuum - the first signs of ADHD

Sleep is when we make and replenish energy stores, such as ATP and glycogen. Sleep fragmentation disrupts this and leaves the child low energy, and their blood filled with catecholamines. This is often seen manifested as poor attention and hyperactivity and it is not uncommon to have children diagnosed with ADHD. As Catalano notes "If enough time passes without healthy sleep, you can see issues like delayed cognitive development, stunted physical growth, and abnormal upper and lower jaw development. The latter ultimately leads to orthodontic and dental problems".

Kalaskars 2021 paper in the Journal of paediatric Dentistry found that Children with ADHD or sleep disturbances should always be assessed for the presence of mouth breathing. Early identification and correction of mouth breathing may help in preventing unnecessary exposure to medication for treating ADHD.

This is a big statement, and sadly one that is not gaining enough societal traction. We appear to be hellbent on treating the difficult child, not hunting for why they are distressed. ADHD diagnosis has continued to significantly rise in the population, with a noted 36% increase in adult diagnosis and 18% in youth, with a big jump in female diagnosis in the decade since 2012[lxxxvi]. I will bluntly point out we have a strong penchant to view this as a psychological (think intangible) or cultural occurrence[lxxxvii], and not as a physical problem with a physiological treatable cause and solution.

Jaw and facial maldevelopment URAS and Apnoea

Along with tongue tie/oral fascial restriction and mouth breathing, there are several causes of sleep apnoea, and other factors such as obesity, age, and cranial maldevelopment issues will also contribute to the development of the condition.

There is some evidence to suggest that orthodontic treatment may be beneficial for people with sleep apnoea. This is because orthodontic treatment can help to correct misaligned teeth and jaw issues, which may contribute to the development or worsening of sleep apnoea. Therefore, orthodontic treatment, such as braces or retainers, help to correct these issues, improving the alignment of the jaw and teeth, potentially reducing the severity of sleep apnoea.

For example, a misaligned bite, jaw, and teeth may cause the airway to become narrowed or blocked during sleep, leading to sleep apnoea, now this is not just due to MTHFR issues and central line cartilage growth dysfunction from an epigenetic effect.

We eat junk so our face has become junk?

Unsurprisingly, since the agricultural revolution we have seen significant jaw shrinkage in the human population, leading to an epidemic of crooked teeth, a lack of adequate space for the last molars (wisdom teeth), and constricted airways, ending as a major cause of sleep-related stress.

The speed with which human jaws have changed, especially in the last few centuries, is much too fast to be evolutionary nor genetic. The changes correlate strongly with phenotypic responses to a vast natural experiment, the rapid and dramatic modifications of our environment.

The agricultural and industrial revolutions have produced smaller jaws and less-toned muscles of the face and oropharynx, which contribute to the serious health problems mentioned above. This is perhaps best demonstrated in the breeding patterns of dogs such as the pug or boxer, who are renowned for poor breathing issues and snoring. Humans in the western world live much more pampered lives, with less physical activity, less threat, with much softer food, that is highly processed and requires little in the way of chewing, much of it you can slurp through a straw, such as yoghurt or jelly, or the, so very popular "smoothie". This starts in early childhood with the introduction of pureed baby foods, which do not exist in nature, the closest likelihood of this is in hunter gatherer societies when the parents pre-chewed food for their weaning infants, but nowhere else did we find pulped food until the industrial revolutions.

The mechanism of change lies in orofacial posture, the way people now hold their jaws when not voluntarily moving them in speaking or eating and especially when sleeping. The critical resting oral posture has been disrupted in societies no longer hunting and gathering. Virtually all aspects of how modern people function, and rest are radically different from those of our ancestors.

Industrialised humanity has developed an unprecedented lifestyle, which has led to our decline. Our lifestyle has dramatically changed the environments in which human beings develop and has led to serious health problems[lxxxviii] including the overlooked jaw developmental issues connected with human jaws.

Orthodontic Dentistry- Profiteer or Saviour?

Dentistry, and largely one branch of it, namely orthodontics, has profited from the decline in oral functional development, and seems to ignore causation of the issue in favour of continued business growth. They continue to profit and have many children wearing braces and then retainers to manage malocclusion no heed of cause, just an offhand "its genetic" or an acceptance of that's just how kids are these days. They treat the symptom of our continuum of dysfunction, not the cause of the issue and the orthodontist continues to kick the symptom down the road.

The prevalence of orthodontic treatment in the United States has increased significantly, by 2009 it was estimated at about 20% of the population. The concern is that orthodontics will be demanded largely for cosmetic reasons, and by the therapist to correct malocclusion, and make a better bite, as necessary improving structure of the upper and lower jaw or improving airway function[lxxxix] . straightening teeth and improving the mesh of the bite, but not the shape of the nasium, nor the length of the mouth structure in many cases, just prettying the crowding the child came in with. Now in fairness orthodontics has progressed and improved its focus since mine was performed in the 80's. I had a posterior tongue tie which was missed in my initial orthodontic work up, and a whole lot of pain from the practice, but my bite still looks pretty if over deep. Current results may not be quite as bad, with expansion plates being more common to try to alter the roof shape and structure, and teeth pulling not as common, however as I noted previously, you're only playing with 10% of the structural cards if this is attempted at 12 years or older, thus the results will never be optimal. We must intervene earlier, preferentially with screening for airway issues in the first year of life.

First Principles • 111

Malocclusion example that are commonly seen

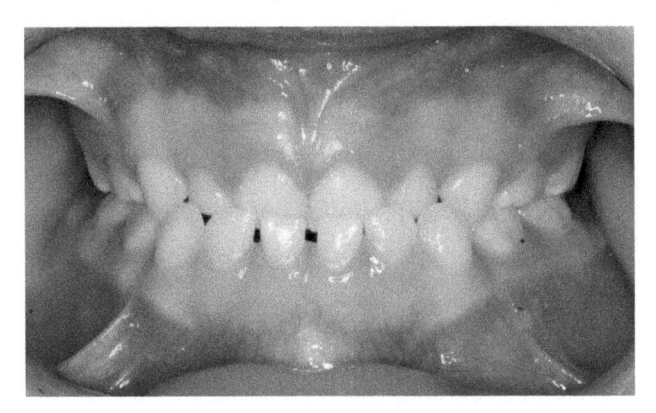

Image 18: The above image demonstrates an anterior cross bite. Note the lower teeth in front of the upper teeth. This will require palette expansion, both to improve biting, and chewing, but also consider the retrusion that the short upper structure causes the tongue.

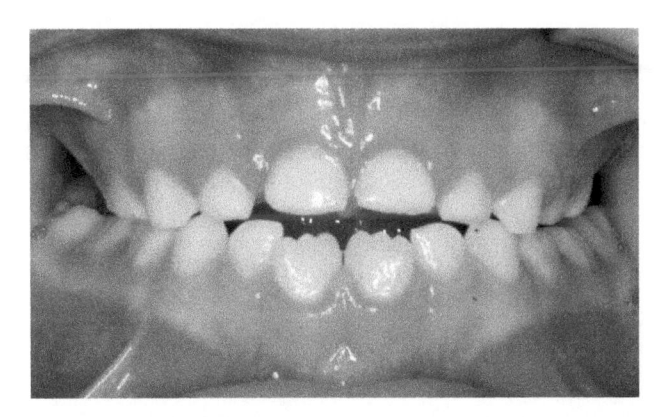

Image 19: The above image demonstrates an Anterior open bite. Note the beak-shaped middle mouth, we see this a lot with bottle feeding, dummy, and thumb sucking. There is also a degree of posterior crossbite with the upper and lower molars not meeting appropriately.

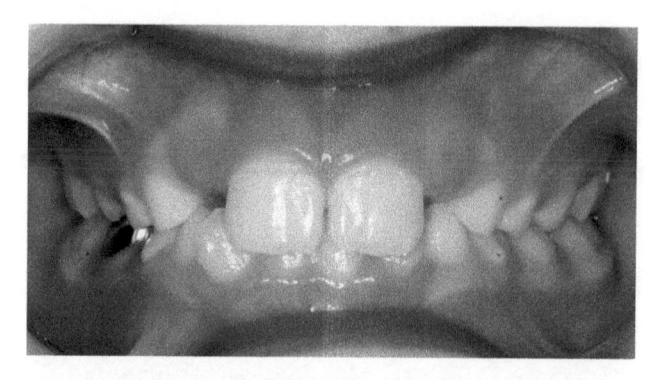

Image 20: The above image is a deep bite. Note the significant covering of the upper adult teeth over the lower teeth. There is also a stainless-steel crown on the lower molar, indicating trauma and intervention has occurred.

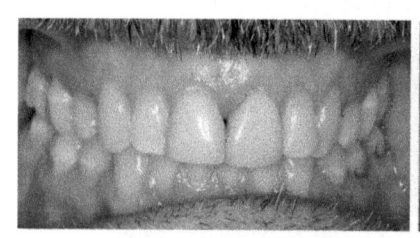

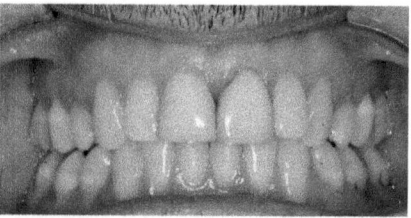

Image 21 and 22: The above images demonstrate the before image (20) of a deep bite on an adult, and the same person 6 months later after using a splint to improve position.

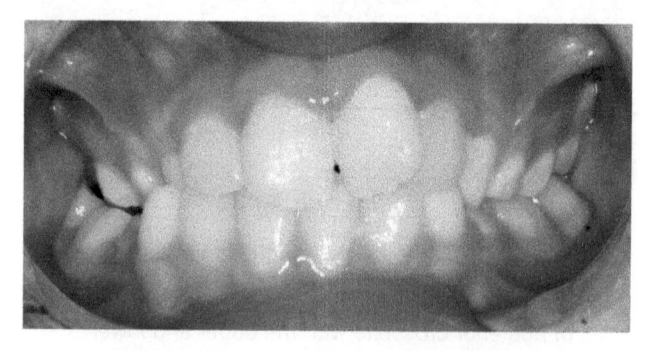

Image 23: The above image shows a Posterior Crossbite with dental crowding and a canted maxilla. The midline structures do not line up and the posterior teeth have been moved sideways and do not mesh with their appropriate lower structure.

It is therefore possible that orthodontic treatment could actually exacerbate UARS and sleep apnoea in some cases. This is because orthodontic treatment, such as braces or retainers, will cause changes to the alignment of the teeth, jaw and maxilla that could narrow or block the airway. This will be most concerning during sleep when respiratory drive decreases. In my own case of orthodontics, without explaining long term repercussions the orthodontist, removed my four premolars, and realigned my bite, setting me with a very high deep arch, and foreshortened my face.

This decrease in longitudinal length of the palette also decreased the space further that my tongue had to sit, exacerbating poor tongue posture. Of note I started to suffer migraines soon after having braces. The literature makes it abundantly clear of the link between migraines, sleep disorders, especially in REM phase sleep, bruxism, and the brain stem[xc] relationships. While I can't say precisely that the orthodontics did it, the link makes sense. We can consider that the airway was likely narrowed with poor tongue posture to start, braces exacerbate the narrowing of the arch, leading to poor night-time breathing and hypoxia. Frequent morning headaches or awakening with headaches are common symptoms in people with OSA and are directly linked to hypoxemia and hypercapnia[xci]. Hypercapnia being defined as an elevation in the arterial carbon dioxide tension.

Orthodontics generally are associated with an increase in pain especially in the early course of treatment, which I certainly experienced, especially from wearing a night-time head brace. Pain is a noted bidirectional disturber of sleep[xcii], thus the increase of pain may have disturbed my sleep as well, potentiating migraine, notwithstanding the strain on the bone of the anterior cranial vault and meningeal structures from the braces themselves. Please remember from our earlier discussion how all cranial bones are interconnected and one cannot apply force to a single unit and not affect the whole. While the brain has no pain receptors, the cranial vault and especially the meninges are packed with nociceptors.

In this whole cycle, we also know that hypoxia is a potent inducer of pain and migraine, and when the situation becomes chronic, windup, and central sensitisation can give the migraine a life of its own. This is another doom loop, the more the brain suffers pain, the more sleep disturbed, which creates fatigue and a greater likelihood of central sensitisation, which combined with mouth breathing and hypercapnia increases the likelihood of a migraine occurring. Further let's draw attention to the brainstem as per Vgontzas work, where we note that issues in the brainstem-cortical networks involved in sleep physiology are important factors in the common migraine pathway. Recent discoveries suggest the hypothalamus as a key mediator in the pathophysiology of migraine, while signalling molecules such as serotonin and dopamine point to a common pathophysiology manifesting in migraine and sleep problems.[xciii]

There is also an increase in people suffering facial and temporomandibular joint pain in our society. This can occur for several reasons but most obviously I believe it is because of clenching of the jaw in defence of airway patency. Commonly called Bruxism, this is termed the involuntary grinding of teeth in the night and is placed in a similar category of involuntary movement as restless leg syndrome (also associated with sleep disturbances apnoea, hypopnea, and migraine). This presumes that there is no rational reason for the muscle activation, that it is not done on purpose to maintain airway, that it has no common pathway behind the occurrence, especially in relation to the pathophysiology of apnoea, migraine, pain and other health issues. The activation of the clench reflex, lifts the hyoid bone, elevates the tongue out of the throat, tightens the pharyngeal muscles, opening the airway while also thrusting the head of the mandible into the articular surface of the mandibular fossa. This compresses the articular disc, in some cases splitting it. There is a strong correlation of bruxism with temporomandibular joint dysfunction (TMD) is known to be a comorbidity with migraine, making it a particularly frequent complaint among patients with migraine. This jaw posturing from the bruxism, also thrusts the head forward, rotating it on its axis, tightening suboccipital muscles and increasing anterior head carriage and the possibility of cranial tenderness and pain.

Studies of sleep bruxism often speak about generalised headaches, as against Migraines along with TMD issues and orofacial pain. Although a well-recognized association, the aetiology of the bruxism-migraine relationship is less well understood. It is possible that bruxism and TMD trigger migraine attacks through increased peripheral activation of the trigeminal nerve, or that patients with migraine are more susceptible to pain from TMD secondary to central sensitization. Lastly, the same central aetiologies proposed for sleep bruxism may possibly directly contribute to migraine, patients suffer with sleep microarousals, and interruptions involved in sleep stage transitions, failure to maintain REM sleep, failure to maintain patent airway leads to hypoxia and a shift in the blood acidity creating a pain windup loop centrally, especially as we have already noted the hypoxic effect on increased immune activation and cytokine production such as IL6.

The innervation to the temporomandibular joint is by branches from the mandibular division of the trigeminal nerve (CN V3), mostly through the auriculotemporal branch, along with branches from the masseteric and deep temporal nerves. The articular tissues and the dense part of the articular disc have no nerve supply. The significance of this situation is that hypoxia is a potent activator of dorsal horn neurons as well as mechanical and thermal hypersensitivity inducting neuropathic pain, thus the hypopnea/apnoeic situation alone can increase pain sensitisation in the patient, globally not just in the TMJ[xciv].

Malocclusion and facial pain are only the tip of the iceberg when considering symptoms of this widespread serious underlying pandemic in the western world. Children are not only suffering with malocclusion and facial pain but are increasingly walking around with poor lip seals, mouth open, as well as sleeping with their mouths open, they are snoring, have upper airway resistance syndrome (UARS), which is leading them to become adults suffering obstructive sleep apnoea.

As previously mentioned OSA refers to having repeated stressful episodes of interrupted sleep from a temporary cessation of breathing, this is often because the subjects' jaw is too small to house the tongue adequately. UARS is sleep fragmentation, often accompanied by snoring, without apnoea, often traceable to narrowed jaws[xcv], and clinically recognisable in children, which leads to other health consequences. Currently the frequency of UARS has not been established, but it seems reasonable to assume that it is higher than the frequency of obstructive sleep apnoea.

Symptoms of Oral Fascial Restriction and tongue tie Adults

Tongue tie symptoms in adults may be like those found in kids. But in adults, a tongue-tie may have progressed to cause a broader set of symptoms, conditions, and diseases. Many of these signs are diagnosed by themselves as stand-alone conditions and are not connected to the underlying pattern. This piecemeal approach commonly leaves the patient not significantly better off;

they continue to evolve more pain and dysfunction. The below list is long but not exhaustive and may include problems that the reader may be aware of but not why it is occurring:

- Daytime Drowsiness
- High blood pressure
- Heart attack
- Stroke
- Atrial Fibrillation
- Type two Diabetes
- Weight gain
- Metabolic disease
- Depression
- Memory loss
- Car accidents
- **Premature Death**
- TMJ Pain
- Dental issues and the need for Crowns
- Orthodontic requirements as a Teenager
- Snoring
- Headaches
- Migraine
- Visual Dysfunction
- Sinusitis
- Sleep apnoea/hypopnea
- Low Energy
- Brain Fog/fatigue
- Digestive dysfunction
- Food Cravings/Sugar hunting

Many of these signs are significant, and not always obvious but all make sense when you consider them for a moment, including those we have already talked about. My favourite in the list is

Premature Death. Because generally we consider, diagnose, and treat the above list as individual conditions, as against as part of a progressive continuum we don't see the links between them all.

We don't see how things like the hypopneas, and apnoea increase intravascular pressure, that the hypoxia increases immune activation, leading to EGRF narrowing arteries and increased blood thickening due to inflammation, that this is all associated with metabolic syndrome, the links to drive dementias and weight gain, regardless of the chronic pain and cracked teeth from jaw clenching.

As noted, IL6 is released due to sleep fragmentation, IL6 can alter serotonin production and function in the brain and can lead to depressive tendencies, anxiety disorders and neurocognitive dysfunction. The fatigue alone leads to brain fog, and all of these reasons give rise to the drive to hunt for a sugar hit to keep going. Which creates another doom loop pushing blood sugar up, insulin up, leading to midbody weight gain, metabolic dysfunction and diabetes, obesity, and inflammation, which then aggravates sleep leading to worsening of the sleep fragmentation and potentiating the loop.

Lip seal issues due to vanity

An interesting point to think about is the new practice of lip augmentation and its possible effects on health. Theoretically the trout pout may give a great capacity for seal in people with poor soft tissue function or maldeveloped skeletal structure, however after observing some of the treated populace, enhancement can leave the patient unable to properly activate the orbicularis oris muscle, which is essential for appropriate lip seal. This is termed Dynamic muscle discord (DMD)[xcvi]. This imbalanced activity between the various facial muscle groups can affect the posture and profile of mobile facial features at rest, think therefore about the effect on sleeping mouth posture and what happens if the lips fall apart while asleep, hint you mouth breath. Unfortunately, despite being a condition that commonly presents in varying degrees in patients seeking lip enhancement, DMD is poorly diagnosed, however it is frequently observed in patients with facial, skeletal, and soft tissue deficiencies. The lack of adequate structural support results in compensatory muscle hypertonicity and can confer a mechanical advantage in certain muscles over their antagonistic counterparts leading to a worsening in function. Ultimately this could lead to mouth breathing and all the problems associated that lead on from it.

Maybe leaving our lips alone and not emulating "The Real Housewives of" wherever is in your best interest if you want to sleep with good lip seal.

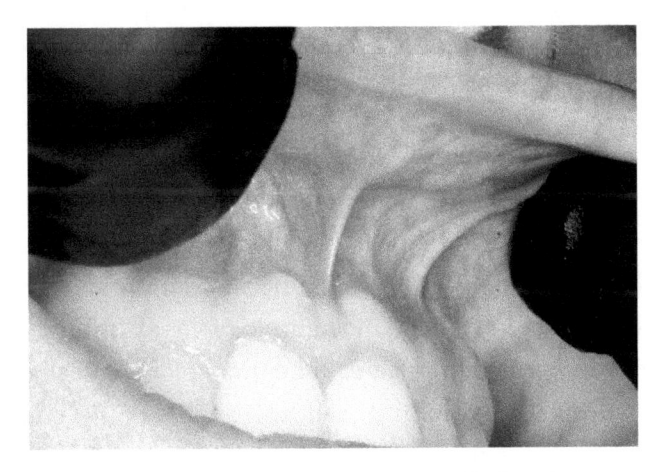

Image 24: Before image of the upper lip frenulum before reduction surgery.

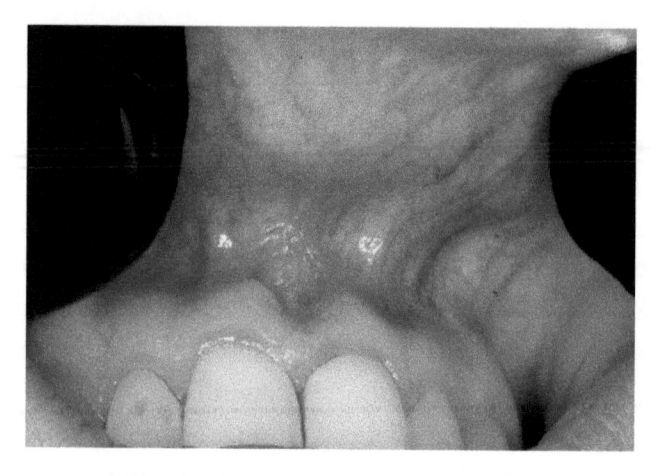

Image 25: The same Lip after the frenulum reduction surgery to allow greater lip movement and improve lip seal.

Neurological Consequences or Causes of Mouth Breathing, Tongue Tie, and Cranial Maldevelopment

HERE WE WILL DETOUR into the neurological aspects of the child's development the following chapters are to try to give the reader an understanding of what is going on at the same time as the skeletal and soft issue is developing issue and how they form a chicken or egg scenario that really can't be separated or effectively determined. It is a primer and not an exhaustive treatise on the involvement of neurology in all things human, that is beyond my scope here. The first place we shall draw attention to is the primitive reflexes as they are commonly ignored and are significant in the interplay from at least 5 weeks in utero through till perhaps 4 years of age if all develops normally, and lifelong if you don't. They are essential for all development and have significant interplay with all of the cranio-facial and respiratory development, and drive the child to develop cortical, neuro-emotional maturity.

By understanding the primitive reflexes and what occurs when they become stuck and unintegrated, we can view the why of a disfunction, and consider how best to help the infant, child, or adult, not just label them into a convenient bucket. In my view the brain is everything and the structure and function is an end result of development around the survival of the brain, thus any deviation from normal brain or nervous system development change's function form and survival capabilities of the resulting organism as we shall discuss.

We will discuss the primitive reflexes largely from the infant and child's perspective and discuss the signs of non-integration, but please be aware that if you can find the reflex in the adult it means that there is a problem. It has either become disinhibited indicating pathology or it never fully integrated, suggesting a developmental problem of the continuum of issues potentially associated with tongue tie, oral facial maldevelopment, airway issues and sleep fragmentation and should elicit a response of investigation of these areas after life threatening pathology has been dismissed. If issues in these areas persist, the brain stays in defensive wind-up loops and integration of the reflex will be largely impossible.

As a final point before we dive in, none of these neurological reflexes nor the physical development of the child's body occur in a discrete packets, one after the other, even though we talk about them as such, nothing occurs in a vacuum, things occur simultaneously and in sliding time zones, overlapping or not depending on the stimuli presented and epigenetics, so no description of when is exact.

7

The Primitive Reflexes:

The following chapter is a discussion of neurological development driven by the hardwired reflexes built into the foetus's Central nervous system (CNS). These "Primitive Reflexes" drive the development of the entire nervous system, enhancing maturation and increased complexity. They are there for a specified time and theoretically no longer. The purpose of Primitive Reflexes is to allow survival of the infant and promotes maturity, myelination, and development of the child to become a functional adult, out of its beginning as a reflexogenically driven learning machine.

If we keep in mind that function drives form, then abnormal function of the primitive reflexes will drive the structure of the developing child to deviate from the theoretical perfect form led to pathology developing in stages across the life of the child.

The below is to bring to the reader's attention several of the important Primitive reflexes that allow development when they appear and should disappear, what their purpose is and when dysfunction occurs what this will look like, the evidence supporting them and ideas about what they become diagnosed as when picked up at an older age of the child/adult. Part of the point of describing them to the reader is to point out these are all reflexes that are capable of being assessed in any bedside exam, by a Paediatrician, a chiropractor, physical therapist, of general practitioner anywhere, that they are currently not commonly checked speaks volumes as to the decline in our examination skills, or the time paucity to assess the patient.

Reflex- A definition

A reflex is an involuntary muscle movement in response to a stimulus to a receptor, such as a stretch receptor in the knee tendon, causing the lower limb to jerk out and back.

As a significant point:

Assessing primitive reflexes may cause undue stress in the infant especially in relationship to the fear paralysis reflex, the Startle and Moro reflexes and should only be used for gaging progress. Repetitive activation of them may hardwire inappropriate responses in the Childs CNS. Please note that it is unadvisable to assess primitive reflexes unless you have been trained by a professional.

The Primitive reflexes are involuntary motor responses hardwired into the brainstem and spinal cord which start during pregnancy are present at birth or soon after. Primitive reflexes are essential in the early development of the new-borns brain and facilitate survival, especially straight after birth, as well as progression towards adulthood. The search, sucking, rooting, and swallowing reflexes which enable breast feeding in the instantly newborn are great examples.

They help the child develop, breathing and feeding ability, spacial awareness, the ability to use hands as tools as well as driving the vestibular system which in due course the development of will allow the capacity to walk upright as well as many other capacities.

These initial central nervous system motor responses are usually inhibited between 4 to 6 months of age as the brain matures and replaces them with voluntary motor activities and postural reflexes, but primitive reflexes may return with the presence of neurological disease such as stroke or from brain injury such as blunt force trauma, or anoxia from drowning[xcvii].

Several reflexes are important in the assessment of new-borns and young infants and will be assessed below. In children the persistence retention of primitive reflexes past 6 months is indicative of developmental delay and may also suggest cerebral palsy and/or neurological damage, especially if five or more abnormal reflexes persist. The adult re-emergence of primitive reflexes indicates decompensation backwards own the developmental landscape and can indicate the potential for several brain pathologies. This is known as frontal release signs, can be seen in the normal adult population. Multiple frontal release signs observed on neurological examination correlate with frontal lobe brain pathology, including Alzheimer disease, multiple sclerosis, and schizophrenia. Therefore, it is important to know how to assess the reflexes in any aged patient.

Fear Paralysis Reflex

One of the first reflexes to appear as part of a neurological development symphony beginning to take shape in the growing foetus is the Fear Paralysis Reflex (FPR). In my opinion, this may be the most important of the primitive reflexes if retained. It appears to set the stage for many other areas of development, and if maintained, it is associated with issues in emotional regulation, ocular, vestibular, and midline muscle function, as well as oral dysfunction starting in the newborn and potentially persisting to later stages of life.

The FPR appears at five to seven weeks in utero, which is exactly the same time as the tongue, and oral structural development in the foetus. This raises the question about who dysfunctions first or whether there is a unifying teratological issue that alters the development of both the oral structure/function and the CNS thus the FPR at this point of the pregnancy. The FPR developmentally is followed by the Moro reflex.

The Moro reflex will be discussed in detail later in the chapter, appears between nine and twelve weeks. This presumes that the FPR begins to integrate and develops into the Moro reflex. The FPR should fully integrate by the twelfth week and therefore be extinguished. Although there are papers that suggest the FPR when integrating transforms into the controller of REM sleep.

The FPR, designed to appear first and integrate first, should not remain active. If it does, the Moro reflex may remain active as well. Similarly, if the Moro is retained, the FPR may not have fully completed its integration.

Any disruption in this early tango of the FPR and the Moro reflex carries the risk of adversely affecting the integration of all the remaining primitive reflexes and altering the development and progression to a functional adult CNS. This can lead to numerous physical, mental, and emotional challenges, which can persist throughout the individual's lifetime, such as OCD, anxiety, or poor emotional attachment.

This makes the FPR and its integration the essential basis for all later development and it gives the capacity for tertiary level emotions and relationships., not just primary level survival behaviours.

The FPR plays a protective role for both the mother and unborn child. It performs the essential, protective task of reducing the demands the foetus places on mums' system as she responds to the danger when encountering a threat with a flight or fight response.

The FPR accomplishes this by causing the foetus to experience immediate motor paralysis, restricted peripheral blood flow, and a lowered heart rate. As a result, more of the mother's physiological resources are partitioned and available for her to respond to the situation. At the same time the FPR protects the foetus by reducing exposure to and absorption of the stress hormones cortisol and adrenaline across the placenta which will be pumping around the mother's blood stream to help her respond to the threat.

If the threat to the developing foetus are toxic chemicals from exposure in the mum's blood stream such as alcohol, then this will activate the FPR's protective action and lessen the foetus's absorption of these agents. Thus, the FPR can function as an automatic reaction to sensory, physical, or psychological stimuli. Imagine therefore the effects of a mother chronically wracked with unrelenting anxiety during the pregnancy upon the FPR activation and the potential alteration in the infants nourishment and development, both physically and cognitively, its highly likely the threat set point of the child will be altered post-partum, let alone consequences to all physiological structures, as discussed previously due to the epigenome or nutritional partitioning away from the foetus to the mother.

Fear paralysis, as its name suggests causes an immobilising fear combined with a significant decrease in heart rate, respiration, and muscle tone, this resembles the phase 4 reptilian response of freeze[xcviii]. The FPR interplays and can control the parasympathetic nervous system, of which the vagus nerve is strongly connected. The vagus nerve is responsible for the regulation of internal organ functions, such as digestion, heart rate, and respiratory rate, as well as vasomotor activity, and certain reflex actions, such as coughing, sneezing, swallowing, and vomiting.[xcix] This association is important, as the vagus nerve can become entrapped in the neck or torso especially by fascia or over tight asymmetric muscles. When this occurs, release of this entrapment by a chiropractor or osteopath may facilitate integration of a retained FPR in the older patient.

The integration of the FPR before birth is important, in part because it supports the child's emotional attachment to parent and leads to social maturity. A child with a poorly integrated FPR may face lifelong anxiety, chronic fears, and even panic disorders. Furthermore, persistence of the reflex after birth can lead to developmental and movement challenges.

A retained FPR may lead to respiratory arrest, heart arrhythmias, and epilepsy/seizures. In addition, there is a possible link to sudden infant death syndrome (SIDS)[c], which occurs mainly at about two to four months of age. These possibilities make sense due to the vagal connection[ci], dysfunction of the FPR could lead to maladaptive performance of the vagus nerve and the thus the organs connected by it, not operating effectively. Birger Kaada[cii] suggests than an FPR reaction (when retained) might be able to affect the nervous system strongly enough to cause a decrease in heart activity, combined with apnoea, which can lead to SIDS. Of note the FPR is not meant to be occurring past birth and could be why the vagal nerve maturation was defective.

In SIDS infants, more small and fewer large myelinated vagal fibres were found than in controls, suggesting that the vagus nerve in infant SIDS victims is relatively immature. This together with delays in central nervous system myelination and dendritic development, indicates neural developmental delay in SIDS kids[ciii], which correlates with the FPR retention.

Infants have also been shown to have an increased risk of SIDS when the mother smokes before, during, or after pregnancy[civ], or if she is exposed to second-hand smoke while pregnant. Tobacco Smoking is known to be an activator of the FPR response[cv]. It is known to have a significant negative impact on the development of nervous structures, neurotransmission, and cognitive functions, and promotes the development of neurodegenerative diseases[cvi].

An Interesting theory relating to FPR and SIDS is how REM sleep developed.

We now consider REM an integral part of the human sleep cycle and the neurological substrate most consistently associated with dreaming and the psychological state. This thesis suggests, REM sleep evolved out of a primordial defensive reflex: tonic immobility. This reflex, sometimes called death-feigning or animal hypnosis, is usually the last line of defence against an attacking predator. Tonic immobility, common in both vertebrates and invertebrates, has a number of neuroanatomical and behavioural attributes that overlap with those of REM sleep. This overlap is suggestive of an evolutionary kinship[cvii]. This theory may suggest the reason why SIDS occurs mainly in REM phase of sleep.

At the cortical and subcortical level, REM sleep has as its hallmarks a desynchronization of the cortical electroencephalogram, similar to that in wakefulness, and pontogeniculo-occipital waves (characteristic electrical potentials generated in the midbrain and pons). Two REM sleep-specific phenomena occur at the motoneuronal level: a strong suppression of postural muscle tone (atonia) and intermittently generated flurries of activity (phasic events), manifested by rapid eye movements, muscle twitches, and increments or decrements in the activity of those muscles not rendered completely atonic. Thus, during REM sleep, excitatory and inhibitory phasic events are superimposed on a tonic cortical activation and motor inhibition.

The REM sleep-specific phenomena are expressed not only in postural but also in respiratory muscles. Upper airway muscle tone is suppressed in parallel to the atonia of postural muscles. This loss of tone is greater than that seen during other phases of sleep and more profound than the depression of respiratory pump muscle (such as the diaphragm and intercostal muscles) activity. Obviously, the respiratory pump muscles should not all become completely atonic, or breathing would cease, which may be exactly the problem. However, complete atonia may occur in some upper airway muscles, one function of which is to secure upper airway patency[cviii]. Thus, we know that there is atonia to the upper airway with poor postural control and an underdeveloped Vagal nerve and brainstem neuronal pool all occurring with dysfunction in the FPR which should have integrated to the Moro reflex and regulate chest muscle and breathing reflexogenic function.

Placing baby on its tummy may inhibit the chest from expanding, reducing the flow of oxygen to the lungs, while laying the baby on its back may give more space for the chest to expand and allow a freer release of the Moro reflex, whose response may also help activate breathing, especially during rem phase of sleep.

The following are the known risk factors for a child developing an unintegrated FPR:

- Heavy smoking, alcohol consumption, drug addiction, and medications during pregnancy
- C-section delivery, highly stressful pregnancy, premature birth, small birth weight
- Sudden infant death syndrome (SIDS) in siblings
- Panic disorders, agoraphobia, or emotional distress in parents

If an infant has a retained FPR, they may exhibit a specific FPR response to a diverse range of sensory and psychological stimuli. These stimuli include restraint of movement; inversion (being turned upside down, affecting the vestibular system); perception of distant movement or shadows; pain; sudden temperature change; smoke (olfactory); separation from mother or familiar environment; and helplessness and hopelessness (generalised anxiety disorder).

As the unintegrated FPR persists from infancy into childhood, the following may elicit hypersensitivity responses; touch, sound, light, smell, and taste; sudden changes in visual field; and vestibular or proprioceptive stimulation. The child may experience tactile hypersensitivity in the form of feeling uncomfortable in clothes or refusing to get dressed, clothes tags may be irritating, or cuffs and collars may be restrictive or threatening. They may panic, exhibit sweating and nausea, and go "white with fear" due to a rapid drop in blood pressure.

Socially, the child may display embarrassment, shyness, or isolation, they may also experience depression, lack of self-belief, and a reluctance to try new activities. Eye contact can be stressful; the decompensation of the CNS is that these children may stare intensely without blinking, with a narrowed field of vision and perception only pertaining to what is immediately in front of them. This alteration of normal eye movements makes sense in the retained **FPR** in an oral dysfunction child, consider what we spoke about. The direction of brain development is tongue and mouth, then up to the eyes then out to the vestibular, all of which are coordinated through the brain stem. If the Neurology of the mouth is disturbed, then the sequence of developed control will become disturbed leading to compensation. Perhaps we need a new lens to view neurodivergent children?

Separation from a loved one/caregiver may elicit the fear response and they can cling to a parent on the first day of school. They may not accept or give affection easily. While some children may exhibit withdrawal, others may overcompensate and manifest aggression. In general, the child has a low stress tolerance, and may exhibit a frozen state or a delayed response when under mental stress or danger. This is commonly viewed as children on the **AUTISM** spectrum. We very well may be neglecting to see points of assessment and intervention in our drive to be accepting and inclusive when the child is viewed through a psychosocial lens not a physiological one.

In the classroom, the child with a retained **FPR** may freeze when confronted with a challenge – reacting rather than responding to a learning opportunity and being disruptive in class, they might give up more easily, withdrawing mentally and physically, including running, they could also require more individual help to learn and be unable to do it without direct support. A general school phobia may be present. Children may try to minimise visibility of the self, to minimise threat to themselves, by speaking softly to avoid being noticed, and can develop fixed classroom routines to survive.

Expressive language disorders are common, including being overcome by emotion, or not responding to classroom discussion or other activities due to shut down, the paralysis response.

FPR children dislike change and show poor ability to adapt. Imagine transitioning from one class to another or from one subject to another in school when your unconscious reflexogenic state is that everything is a threat and induces fear, fight, or freeze. To suggest this is challenging is an understatement, overwhelming seems more fitting. Confrontation avoidance behaviour is common and may include the drive to pacify or please even when this may go against the child's own self-interest. There may be perfectionism and a fear of failure as well as general negativity or a defeatist attitude.

Temper tantrums including breath holding are not out of the question. Phobias and nightmares may also occur as well as panic disorders, general anxiety, or anxiety over trivial matters, it is difficult to calm the hyperactive response.

We continue to see a retained FPR in people diagnosed with autism or autism-like symptoms. This raises interesting questions to whether the retained FPR leads on to the development of Autism or there is another common factor to both. Autism affects social behaviours and communication, attachment, and emotional development, which leads to cognitive development and learning delay in many cases. Children with autism with a retained FPR can display selective mutism. It consists of the inability to speak in certain stressful situations due to temporarily paralysed vocal cords.

As we can see, the retained FPR sets up a discord inside the individual; the manifestations of this are far-reaching and highly varied. Obsessive Compulsive Disorder (OCD) is likely to be related to a retained FPR; so, too, is Attention Deficit

Hyperactivity Disorder (ADHD)[cix]. As the FPR is a heightened stress response it is likely that children and adults with an unintegrated FPR will display eating and sleeping disorders as well.

High blood pressure, shallow or difficult breathing, floppy muscle tone, and tension in the neck and shoulder can all be indicators of the unintegrated FPR, which mirrors the alterations seen in oral fascia tethering and dysfunction. As FPR is a survival mechanism, increased levels of the stress hormones cortisol and adrenaline are released when the reflex is triggered. And there may be a white pallor caused by blood moving to the internal organs, and away from the skin, if this goes on too long it could lead ultimately to a loss of consciousness – the brain's final withdrawal when stress is too hard to endure. In the Adult FPR sufferer we can see this as Postural orthostatic tachycardia (POTS).[cx]

Other physical signs of the FPR is a pigeon-toed foot pattern with the legs turned in, with frustration intolerance. This is a propping mechanism to help support locomotion when the vestibular mechanism is not well integrated, the turned feet is like a snow plough position when skiing and it makes it harder for the individual to fall over as the standing base is wider. All is done on purpose for survival.

As we can see the fear paralysis reflex is super important to human development and is one of the first reflexes to emerge at five to seven weeks in utero. Its initial purpose is to protect mother and child during dangerous times and automatically reduces the metabolic demands the foetus places on the mother's system as she strives to survive. The FPR protects the foetus from absorbing the mother's excessive cortisol, adrenaline, and other toxins by slowing or shutting down its systems. This reflex is scheduled to integrate before birth into the Moro reflex. If unintegrated, we may see associated conditions such as ADHD, autism, central auditory processing disorder, dyspraxia, obsessive-compulsive disorder, and selective mutism.

Signs the Fear Paralysis Reflex may not be fully integrated:

- Decreased stress tolerance
- Oversensitivity of the senses (eyes, ears, touch, smell, taste)
- Motion Sickness
- Difficulties with eye contact
- Temper Tantrums and acting out behaviour
- Obsessive Compulsive symptoms
- Oppositional and aggressive behaviour
- Withdrawal and Elective mutism
- Excessive shyness

Moro Reflex

The Moro reflex is an essential developmental neurological reflex referred to as the "gateway" reflex, as its development from the FPR is essential to pave the way for other reflexes that contribute to survival and learning, while also helping to create movement and cognition in all other later aspects of life. Originally given the name of "Umklammerungreflex" (embracing or clasping reflex)[cxi] by Moro, who likened its use as essential for holding onto mother when both are under duress as seen by orangutans in nature and a tiger appears, his name stuck, and the mouthful did not.

The Moro reflex should appear at nine to twelve weeks in utero progressing on from and helping to integrate the FPR, according to some for the rest of our lives, that when successfully accomplished, allows the Moro reflex to emerge and the FPR to exit the CNS and lay the foundation for all the reflexes to follow, and avoid many of the previously mentioned dysfunctions. The consequences when the dance is not accomplished allows the FPR to continue and alter the set point of the CNS and emotional state of the child for life.

The integration of the Moro reflex itself, is designed to occur three to four months after birth, by six months as the outlier. The harmonisation between the Moro reflex and its early partner the FPR sets the tone for the successful development of all the subsequent reflexes.

The neural centre of the Moro reflex seems located in the lower part of the brain, specifically the brainstem because this reflex is present in anencephalic new-borns (Karlsson,1962).

Vestibular stimulation plays a crucial role in triggering the Moro reflex with experiments fixing the head and body of the child on a table or a tilting chair to remove any proprioceptive stimulation of the muscles of the neck (Prechtl, 1965), and, in anencephalic infants, it was only obtained when the vestibular nuclei were preserved (Hanabusa, 1975). This gives the indication of which systems will be affected by incomplete integration of the reflex, also suggesting the location of the Moro reflex is the Colliculus.

From this we know that the Moro is involved with head position in space and entraining head righting, and head and eye movement to a target.

The Moro reflex plays a protective role for the developing infant. It produces an automatic response to sudden stimuli such as loud noises, changes in lighting, movement in the visual field, or tactile contact. The Moro reflex guards the infant who has not yet developed higher brain centres to understand the world thus a physical reaction is given by reflex to stimulus.

In a study of 13 new-borns, all Moro reflexes occurred after a Startle reflex. This association suggests that the Moro reflex could also be controlled like the Startle reflex by the FEAR system and can therefore be understood as an active defence behaviour of the flight, fight, freeze system in the human new-born who cannot move and replaces fleeing by a gesture of communication to its human environment[cxii].

As noted, the Moro reflex contributes to the development of the child before, during, and after birth. It gives protective abilities to the underdeveloped child and helps develop the breathing mechanism and coordinate the suck, swallow, breath reflex[cxiii] and provides the energy and adrenaline to begin the birthing process and help swim down the vaginal canal. It helps the newborn take its first breath, opening the lungs. The Moro reflex triggers extension of the newborn's body which has been largely flexed in the "foetal position" for the entire pregnancy. The Moro reflexes drive development to maintain horizontal and vertical head position as well as sitting and standing without support (in later childhood) due to its connections to the vestibular mechanism.

After birth, the Moro's protects the child reflexively in two distinct phases: in the first phase, the Moro reflex causes the baby to arch the head back, lift the arms up and back, spread the fingers, and take a gasp of air and hold it. This is considered an avoidance response to possible danger.

In the second phase, the Moro reflex causes the child to curl forward, pull the legs up, fold the arms across the chest, clench the fists, and breathe out and cry for help.

This phase involves a grasping response, which enables the child to cling to (presumably) the mother and help the child avoid a fall. By curling forward, they can protect the soft squishy underbelly or more vulnerable parts of the body and the face.

There is a significant association between the occurrence of the Moro reflex and the placement of the new-born at birth on the mother's abdomen; the research had a p value = 0.002 meaning that there was no way it could be by chance. The researchers found that there was no association of the moro reflex with maternal primiparity, prenatal stress, Group B streptococcus carriers, agitation during delivery, new-born's gender, labour induction, epidural anaesthesia, foetal scalp electrode placement, and full versus half-light in the delivery room, only the placement on the mother in a supine vs lateral position.[cxiv] This is suggestive of the reflex having a strong survival function, it gives connection to mother, holding to the body and allows for feeding response. This then drives the aforementioned up eyes movement, back and neck extension.

Rousseau's paper takes our thinking in an important different direction, it brings attention to the magnitude of arm abduction-extension and fingers spreading by the baby, their rigid posture at the highest point of movement, and the stereotyped shape of the movement are features of ritualization which is an evolutionary process of transforming a physiological behaviour into a communication behaviour whose purpose is to improve mutual understanding between individuals of the same species to prevent damaging conflicts and strengthen emotional bonds.

This is a huge concept taking the neonates behaviour from the realm of a pure reflex automation; it is no longer just movement behaviour, but rather a communication stereotype used to activate the maternal behaviour system, and to protect the neonate.

The Moro reflex is designed to integrate into the expanding nervous system and effectively disappear at approximately four to six months of age. After this point, persistence of the reflex can be an indication of neurodevelopmental delays. Of interest as the Moro response diminishes, the Strauss reflex takes over. The Strauss reflex is considered the adult startle response. When stimulated a startled person to put his shoulders up, blink, relax, locate the source of stimulus, and resume activities. The Strauss reflex allows the individual to become habituated to irrelevant sounds and respond to relevant ones. This means, for example, you can filter out unnecessary background noise such as traffic sounds, yet still notice when someone calls out your name. Theoretically the Strauss reflex is appropriate and not just an observation of continued FPR/Moro activity in the CNS. As primitive reflexes are not regularly studied, the body of literature does not readily contain an easily verifiable answer to this question.

Moro Reflex is increasing.

The number of children with retained Moro reflexes appears to be rising in our western populations. This is due to such factors as poor nutrition; environmental contaminants including chemicals, toxins[cxv] , and electromagnetic frequencies; as well as birth stresses, including C-section delivery, forceps births, breach births, and prematurity. As previously noted, birth stresses can create problems that persist throughout childhood and beyond. Illustrating this point a 2015 study demonstrated that 35% of healthy 4-6 years old's examined had significant and persistent retained primitive reflexes along with altered motor and emotional development[cxvi]. In the study over 60% of children demonstrated at least one primitive reflex at level 1–2 and 25% of them at levels 3 and 4, the higher the number the more retained and strongly elicited. This result means that most of the examined pre-school children have non-integrated reflexes[cxvii]. The authors suggested that large scale testing of the normal population of school children would be beneficial, which I agree with, both for the primitive reflexes such as the Moro, as well as for tongue tie, mouth breathing and sleep fragmentation, as well as maldevelopment of the mouth and bite.

When is the Moro is not Normal?

While the persistence of the Moro reflex beyond six months of age can create serious disruption and developmental delays in the growing child, a Moro reflex that is either absent, asymmetrical, or overactive in the child before 6 months of age, is also a matter of concern.

The gravest concern, the Moro Reflex being absent and un-elicitable in the newborn, suggests upper-motor neuron lesions indicating damage to the brain or spinal cord. In the first few weeks of life, absence of the reflex is seen in infants who have been deeply sedated, in those who suffered a severe cerebral insult either prenatally or during birth, and in premature babies.

An asymmetrical Moro reflex as seen by one arm not moving the same as the other or not at all, may indicate hemiplegia (paralysis affecting one side of the body), it could also be a fractured clavicle on the non-activating limb, or suggest Erb's Palsy (paralysis of the arm causes by injury to the brachial plexus in the neck/shoulder). These are all signs of trauma in the neonate and should provoke immediate further medical assessment.

Infants with an overactive Moro reflex, on the other hand, are likely to startle at the slightest sounds and have significant difficulty staying asleep. This is expressed by parents saying they must "walk on eggshells" to keep the room quiet, to avoid startling or waking the newborn. The baby may cry frequently, be clingy and fussy, and be difficult to comfort. While one infant may dislike affection, another may feel insecure and want to be held all the time. This resembles the situation where the FPR has not integrated, interfering with the CNS development. In my experience newborns with abnormal suck swallow breath reflexes, tongue tie and sleep fragmentation will generally have an associated FPR/Moro hyperactivation, which significantly ameliorates with Tie removal and rehabilitation. The Moro is a survival reflex and is hyper-activated when the child's nervous system believes they are significantly under threat and should advise their mother to save them.

Nothing is more threatening to the neonate's survival as an impediment to breathing, acquiring nourishment, or sleeping. They do not thrive in this scenario. Therefore, I suggest that we should view all babies with a hyperactive startle and poor sleep practices as having a physiological issue until proven otherwise and that the actions such as controlled crying and other control parenting practices as inappropriate to the needs of a child who very likely has a physical issue, even if not understood yet. And should be dispensed with until such time as the child has rationality to actually choose to behave poorly such as in toddlerdom, if then.

As the infant develops an unintegrated Moro may cause immature eye movements and visual problems[cxviii], including difficulty ignoring irrelevant visual input[cxix]. Partially this is rooted in the issue of up eye development as discussed earlier in the book, as part of the tongue tie complex hampering brain stem control and development of eye function and alteration of eye preference created by non-optimal feeding practices and posture.

As a result, the child may have difficulty sustaining visual attention. They may find it hard to manage rapidly approaching stimuli, as in the case of catching a ball. In the classroom, the child may find it difficult to focus on details and copy from the black board. In general, Moro retaining children will be more distractible. This statement however doesn't do justice to why a behaviour occurs, it just states that it does occur. By this stage I would hope the reader would have learned that my favourite question is why something is not what. Why is the child's visual field distractible is super important, not just labelling that they have a problem.

Consider it thusly, in reality, the child who has not integrated the Moro/FPR (threat response to stimuli reflex) is assessing the environment for threat, they consider the object of fixation, make a safe not safe decision about it, and move to the next item or perhaps react to it if they determine it resembles a threat. Their unconscious brain doesn't feel safe; therefore, they stay forever vigilant. A good defence is a great offence, see it kill, it asks questions after. They can't attend to an object for very long as once it is coded as low threat they must move to assess or are stimulated to attend to other objects/events in their environment. These FPR/Moro children are constantly looking for threat, which is the basis of anxiety and strongly resembles ADHD, which is also associated with poor sleep patterns and fatigue.

In addition, vestibular challenges such as poor balance and coordination as well as motion sickness may occur as a result of an unintegrated Moro reflex. Consequently, the child may dislike playing, tumbling activities such as gymnastics, or amusement park rides such as a roller-coaster or dodgems.

The unintegrated Moro reflex continues to influence aspects of behaviour as the child develops, even in adulthood, the individual may live in constant stress, with the body going into fight or flight whenever stimulus elicits the reflex. Repeated activation of the reflex causes excess secretion of cortisol and adrenaline, fatiguing the adrenal glands and the brain and hyperactivating the immune system in defence, this leads to the child/adult suffering chronic colds and allergic conditions.

Other characteristics of the unintegrated Moro include cravings for sweets as the body requires more energy to stay on high alert, which is linked to excessive cortisol production, and snacking (inability to eat a whole meal). These individuals may also suffer from headaches.

Poor adaptability and dislike of change is another characteristic of the unintegrated Moro reflex. The individual may have difficulty approaching new situations, choosing instead to withdraw, this is the flight part of the poly vagal response. They may be fearful in social situations, or alternately, may be overbearing and controlling, consider it another defence mechanism. If I control all the parts, it can't hurt me. They may experience generalised insecurity, anxiety, and fear, including panic attacks and mood swings. For children, this may take the form of aggressive outbursts, even hitting, pitching and biting. These children are frequently "picked on" because of these behaviours as well as their tendency to overreact. Both children and adults may have difficulty accepting or giving affection. Successful integration of the Moro reflex is a key element affecting every phase of an individual's lifespan.

Once integration of the Moro begins, the child may experience emotional ups and downs as the nervous and hormonal systems readjust. Considering the consequences of a Moro reflex that is "stuck" or unintegrated, it is imperative to help the child move through this phase, as it is essential for the individual to integrate the Moro to become a functional adult.

An important concept regarding the Moro reflex, is from 2017 paper which proposes that it is a ritualised behaviour of nonverbal communication, rather than a non brain reflex of fear, rather an "asking for help mechanism" left over from infancy that is no longer age appropriate, I like this thought process, however it does not detract from the need to look at mechanisms to help integrate it, or for physiological reasons why it may be active.

Professionals should avoid stimulating the newborns' fear system by unnecessarily triggering Moro reflexes. Antenatal education should teach parents to respond to the Moro reflexes of their newborn infant by picking them up in their arms with motherese talk a sing song prosodic melody type of speech, a cooing at the child if you will that is shown to calm the infant.

In summary, the Moro paves the way for the successful emergence and integration of all the subsequent reflexes. It plays a role in facilitating the birth of the child, protects the infant from excessive or sudden stimuli, and prepares the baby for maintaining vertical and horizontal head position. The absence of the Moro, or its appearance as asymmetrical or overactive, may indicate neurological disorders. A retained Moro is often seen in conditions such as: **ADHD**, autism, central auditory processing disorders, cerebral palsy, dyspraxia, dyslexia, visual processing disorders, along with other neurological conditions and pathologies. Integrating the Moro reflex is essential for a functional CNS in adulthood.

While it is sensible to remind professionals that they should avoid stimulating the new-borns' fear system by unnecessarily triggering Moro reflexes, as it may interfere with normal CNS development and provoke inappropriate hardwiring, It is possible that this concept does not fully describe the purpose of the Moro as a communicative tool and that maybe the trauma has already occurred which has stopped the Moro from integrating, but that this reflex and the child need love and rehabilitation. Antenatal education should teach parents to respond to the Moro reflexes of their new-born infant by picking her up in their arms with mother talk to help soothe it into extinction.

To trigger an active Moro response in an adult or infant, we need to cause a sudden change in the head position in relation to the body, or by a sudden change of body position in space beyond the vertical midline, such as falling back. When the reflex is triggered an increased amount of cortisol and adrenaline is released in the bloodstream, this tightens up muscles including the airway, which may be a physiologic advantage to why it persists in patients with oral fascial structural dysfunction. This has many consequential effects on the patient's physiology including altering immune system function, slower healing, disturbed sleep and increasing disease progression including neuro-emotive imbalance and cognitive issues.

Spinal Galant Reflex

The spinal Galant reflex begins to appear at twenty weeks in utero. This reflex facilitates the development of the anatomy and physiology of the foetus's vestibular and auditory processing system, which begins during the fourth month of gestation. In late pregnancy, it causes inversion of the foetus, creating the proper position for birth. You can therefore imagine that retention of the FPR/Moro reflex might create issues with this reflex operating properly as they strongly affect head position in space and the vestibular collicular mapping.

The Galant reflex is named for the doctor who discovered it, Galant noticed that stroking along the spine of a neonate or a quite young infant, held with its abdomen on his left palm, elicited a characteristic reflex movement. It is rapid and resembles the curving of the body of a lizard as it winds its way rapidly through the grass[cxx]. He elicited it in 150 normal young infants and found it persisted in six out of sixteen epileptic subjects between 7 and 30 years old. He found it was more strongly elicited than the Babinski and persisted longer, by both a stroke of the reflex hammer or pricking the spinal tissue. This was a ground-breaking observation of the nervous system.

The spinal Galant reflex remains active after birth for the first three to six months of an infant's life and should usually integrate during this time. Persistence of the reflex beyond nine months is considered a potential sign of neurological pathology. As noted from the discussion of the previous two reflexes, poor integration of the previous gateway reflexes, The FPR and Moro, may interfere with the appropriate integration of the spinal Galant.

This reflex contributes to the development of the inner ear, enabling hearing and the all-important balance capabilities required by an infant to begin creeping and crawling then onto walking and running at a later age. It supports the development of muscles of the lower back, buttocks, pelvic area, and the back of the legs. The reflex then helps to prepare the infant for standing and walking by assisting in the development of gross motor coordination[cxxi].

The importance of the spinal Galant reflex may be seen in the challenges faced by a child in whom the reflex is retained. When it is retained past the first year of life, a child may have difficulty controlling the legs when walking and running. They may exhibit an unbalanced gait, including impaired hip rotation, leading to self-tripping. As a result, the child may dislike physical activity and sports[cxxii]. If the spinal Galant is retained on one side, the child may develop scoliosis of the spine. Later in life, they may be susceptible to spinal injuries due to the influence of this reflex on L5/S1 joint., the creation of stress on the joint by overactivation of the paraspinal and pelvic muscles.

A child with a retained spinal Galant reflex may exhibit fidgeting and squirming commonly called having as "ants in the pants", when seated in a classroom scenario, which may be due to hypersensitivity to tactile stimulation. Tight clothing, certain textures such as rough wool, and clothing labels may elicit a hypersensitive or ticklish response, especially when a child attempts to sit with his back against a chair. The child often has a preference to do homework or watch television while lying on the floor, so that the reflex is not elicited or aggravated as it would be while seated. Requests for the child to "sit still" or "sit quietly" may cause them to manage his discomfort in other ways, often leading to noise-making in the form of grunting, humming, popping or lip smacking, blowing, and other such sounds.

Not surprisingly, school-aged children with an unintegrated spinal Galant reflex may experience challenges with focus, concentration, and school performance in general. There may be difficulty concentrating on classroom lessons, as the child struggles to comprehend both verbal instructions and written materials. He may exhibit delayed cognition, poor short-term memory, and mental fatigue. ADHD is often present in these children, and there may be impairment in fine motor coordination, notably handwriting[cxxiii].

Other troubling symptoms can be a higher incidence of bed-wetting and soiling of the pants. Sleeping on the back or changing position during sleep may elicit the reflex, triggering the bed-wetting. A second reflex known as the spinal Perez may be a factor here as well.

To elicit the response, one can run the fingers along either side of the spinal column from the base of the neck down to the top of the sacrum. This results in hip flexion in the direction of the stimulus. Sometimes an infant also responds by raising and extending a leg.

Constant supine lying position prevents the integration of the spinal Galant reflex, which therefore if unintegrated can cause bed wetting up until 8-12 years of age.

At about 4 months of age the infant reflexes drive a cross diagonal an eye/hand/foot/mouth movement reflex, if this is not conditioned enough the pathway will not be appropriately myelinated and integrated, leading to long-term consequences for social capacity and interaction in later life. This reflex action sets the spatial awareness for where you start and finish, your personal space, and boundaries.

A major point to remember is that this is not just physical, this sets the aspects of the emotional being as well, Empathy, and the ability to "grasp" how someone else feels is first practised physically. The only difference between thinking "I love you" and saying it is the basal ganglia, inhibiting the motor plan to activate the muscles of the face. Emotions are physical occurrences of the body, not etheric, and like all physical outputs, these require practice to integrate all the motor system, and feedback loops to integrate and make sense of the interna and external world.

To summarise the spinal Galant reflex emerges at about twenty weeks in utero and remains active for the first three to six months of life. It contributes to the development of the inner ear, enabling hearing and the balance required for movement leading to crawling. It supports development of muscles of the low back, buttocks, pelvis, and the back of the legs, then helps to develop gross motor coordination, preparing the child to stand and walk. The spinal Galant when retained, is associated with numerous challenges: difficulty with leg control while walking or running, often leads to a dislike of sports; susceptibility to scoliosis and other spinal abnormalities; hypersensitivity to tactile stimulation that causes fidgeting in class and a preference to lie down instead of sitting during activities; the children can have challenges' with focus, concentration, and school performance; poor short-term memory and often suffer mental fatigue; impairment in fine motor coordination, notably hand-writing; and bed-wetting can also occur.

To trigger the spinal Galant, have the infant or adult laying on their stomach and draw a line from the neck to the sacrum beside the spine over the paraspinal muscles with a fingertip or a reflex hammer tip. This will elicit a sideways flexion from the hip to the ribcage if the reflex is persistent. The leg is also automatically bent into flexion.

Crossed Extensor Reflex

The Crossed extensor reflex (CER) beings in the 28th week of the pregnancy and will remain in action till about the 2nd month postpartum. It becomes integrated into the nervous system and higher brain centres if all goes to plan and will continue to help the child develop.

Also known as leg cross flexion, the crossed extensor reflex is a withdrawal reflex that enables coordinated locomotion and balance, influencing the development of both movements as well as cognitive functions, but only if properly integrated.

The CER allows the foetus to perform kicking actions in the womb. The crossed extensor works in an integration with the ATNR and the stepping reflex to trigger the kicking action, this is a great example of the nervous system developing higher functions.

The CER allows the baby to develop the concept or awareness of having two legs and their position in space. Developing a spatial map with known parts such as head versus neck, versus the trunk which has separate legs and arms positioned in relationship to them is essential for function as a human. The CER is essential for the Thomas automatic gait reflex to develop[cxxiv].

The purpose of the primitive reflexes is to help mature circuits in the brain essential for development and long-term survival, the successful integration of the CER indicates that the medulla oblongata which is in the lower portion of the brainstem is myelinating and is part of the communication loop with higher brain centres.

To get to the essential capacity of being human namely standing and moving on our hind legs the CER causes the development of cross-lateral movement, first crawling then balancing on one leg at a time, which in turn helps to build the corpus callosum that connects the two hemispheres of the brain. A mature corpus callosum that connects the two hemispheres of the brain, will support the coordination of the two hands and feet, binocular vision, and binaural hearing, this means the eyes yoked and the ears working, creating a 360-degree sound scape. Then both sets of sensory organs working together, with balanced core muscles to stabilise the trunk and movement to orientate to stimuli/threat and allow response.

The CER via the corpus collosum enables the limbs to function as a coordinated unit, utilising teamwork, and pairing. To allow locomotion we observe the right leg flexing, while the left leg extends, as this occurs, we see the fore limbs also work in co-ordinated action. As the right leg flexes, the opposite arm also flexes and the right arm extends and let's not forget that the muscles of the trunk contract to stabilise the pelvis and spine/trunk, which will allow walking and running in the future.

The ultimate goal of the CER many years into the future is to help the adult to maintain balance and possibly escape injury or danger this is seen when an individual steps on a sharp object and simply withdraws by jerking the foot back/up, theoretically if all is well, they don't over balance and fall. A complex version of the CER response is seen when an individual is in motion, they extend one leg automatically to maintain balance. This frees the other leg for movement, as in avoiding an oncoming car. In this situation, the first leg briefly extends for balance as the other quickly extends and then flexes to promote forward motion. This movement is triggered as signals move up the spinal column and stimulate the contralateral muscles of the hip and abdomen. As a result, the body's centre of gravity is transferred over the extended leg and the opposite leg is then free to move.

The CER is activated in the infant, by firmly pressing the centre of the sole of the upper foot (the inside of the ball of the foot in the area of K1 which is an acupuncture point) usually with the thumb. As a "contralateral" reflex, a response occurs in the leg opposite to the stimulated foot. The opposite leg will flex, adduct, and then extend again.

A retained or unintegrated crossed extensor reflex is seen after 3 months of age in the infant and can lead to delays in higher nervous system maturation in the cortex and delay in efficient communication between the two brain hemispheres across the corpus callosum.

Retention of the CER can cause delay or abnormality in the infant's concept of having two legs. Think of it as a concept of cortical map smudging, an inability of the brain to find the leg parts separate from each other, and further separate from the trunk, making it hard to localise the individual muscles to move them in a coordinated fashion. This will first be observed in the infant as they begin to try to move independently. This means problems with crawling development. The children may have difficulty moving both legs up and down as well as shifting of body weight side to side. Infants may bum shuffle rather than commando crawl or be unable to coordinate the limbs effectively to make forward motion, frequently pitching forward.

Walking may be asymmetrical in that, one leg crosses in front of the other, or both legs move at the same time in a hopping-like motion, while there is often an active stepping reflex, along with CER that affects walking balance and control in cerebral palsy cases. At this point I would like to note that there are other possible reasons or contributing reflexes for these dysfunctions, including poor integration of the FPR/Moro, as well as trauma to the body.

In some cases, a retained crossed extensor response indicates a disturbance in the corticospinal motor pathway. This disturbance may lead to difficulties with leg coordination, balance, and stability, affecting both body posture/symmetry and muscle development including those of binocular vision. In this case, think about the orchestra of CNS not playing in a coordinated fashion, and the child having several retained reflexes including the FPR, Moro, spinal gallants and possibly issues with myelination.

The end points of these retentions are seen in younger children who may have difficulty with the following: handwriting and other fine motor skills such as buttoning shirts and tying shoes; math difficulties (dyscalculia), especially story problems and multiplication tables; reading, notably related to phonemic awareness; and saccades.

Children may also be seen to exhibit concrete thinking (seeing choices as black or white, an inability to generalise) and diminished general cognitive functions, including speed of perception and thinking.

Children with problems of The CER will benefit from versions of commando crawling to try to drive integration.

Spinal Perez Reflex

The spinal Perez reflex (SPR) begins at the point of baby maturity to help the child be born into the world, this differs from many other primitive reflexes, such as the Moro, which first appear in utero and continue into the first few months of the child's life.

The SPR is elicited with the baby lying in prone position on a hard surface, e. g., an examination table or mattress, or held face down on the examiner's hand. Using moderate pressure, the examiner runs his index finger or thumb along the spine from the pelvis upward to the neck, the opposite direction of the spinal Galant reflex. The baby should lift the head, and arch the back and neck backwards, an infant with a retained SPR may also scream.

In response to this stimulus, Juanico and Pérez list the following reactions:

- Flexion of the lower extremities
- Lordosis of the spine, with elevation of the pelvis
- Flexion of the upper extremities, with elevation of the head
- Strong cry, leading in many cases to glottic spasm with apnoea and occasional cyanosis
- Urination[cxxv].

The SPR is active for the first two to three months of life and helps support the birth process and in the development of movement and mental processing of the infant. Assuming normal development one would expect the baby's cortical pathways to mature significantly from three to six months of age, allowing the spinal Perez reflex to integrate. The SPR can remain active until year two of the infant's life.[cxxvi]

The SPR should integrate and become the Tendon guard reflex and the symmetrical tonic Neck Reflex (STNR) having made important contributions to the infant's development towards maturity. The SPR helps the development of many physical functions of the child including gross motor coordination and symmetrical functioning. Think, walking and running, as well as clapping hands and swimming the overarm stroke, while initially helping the infant expel toxins which remain from the maternal bloodstream as well as activating the baby's Cerebrospinal fluid[cxxvii]. It is protective and sets the basis of body coordination and provides a feeling of positive protection, which may show as low-grade anxiety and worry in a more adult person if poorly integrated.

During the birthing process the SPR coordinates with the asymmetrical tonic neck reflex (see later in book) to stop the labour process to give the child a break.[cxxviii]

If there is an absence of the SPR we must always consider pathology. It could indicate severe cerebral damage from the birth process (think low oxygen supply) or soon after, injury to the upper cervical cord, or severe myopathy. Likewise, the retained reflex carries with it various challenges, ranging from physical to emotional and mental. With a retained spinal Perez, a child may exhibit decreased coordination, muscle tone, and strength. As an adult the individual may experience low back pain and be more likely to have back injuries[cxxix].

The SPR ties in with a retained FPR and can lead to emotional disruption. Emotionally, the child may exhibit instability and be subject to fears and phobias, they may show a lack of impulse control as well as feelings of inadequacy.

The retained spinal Perez reflex affects the development of cognition, psychological health, and social skills. The child may exhibit speech disorders and difficulty expressing information[cxxx] as well as displaying as a narrowed field of vision.

The retained reflex can delay the speed of communication from the brain stem to the midbrain then to the frontal lobes. A retained SPR can also delay the development of the cerebrospinal fluid pumping mechanism and impact the cranial movement system. These delays ultimately affect mental processing speed, memory, logical thinking, and creativity. This may present as focus and concentration difficulties, as well as inability to position and remember objects in space, these characteristics are noted in patients diagnosed with ADHD[cxxxi], giving a direction of care for said patients.

In a similar vein, the retention of the SPR may delay the myelination and thus active functioning of the pineal gland. The Pineal gland is essential to produce melatonin as well as regulation of the circadian rhythm and our ability to count time internally. A disturbance of melatonin production or the circadian rhythm might alter the child's sleep cycle, possibly explaining the relationship of the retained reflex and increased incidents of bed-wetting, which is associated both the retained spinal Perez reflex and the retained spinal Galant reflex. With pineal maturation delayed, bed-wetting may occur because of decreased cortical control during sleep. The retained spinal Galant or spinal Perez can also be stimulated in the lumbar region when shifting positions during sleep or because of pressure from the waistband of elasticated pyjamas. This pressure can also stimulate bed-wetting.

Babinski Reflex

The Babinski reflex or plantar response is a reflex that involves not only the toes, but all muscles that shorten the leg is appears approximately one week after birth[cxxxii]. First described by French neurologist Joseph Babinski in 1896, this reflex remains active during the first year of life and may not completely integrate until the age of two. At that point, it should be extinguished to make way for the appropriate adult flexor response.

To elicit the Babinski reflex, one should stimulate the outside edge of the foot from the heel to the base of the toes. This is performed with a single smooth stroke, light but firm pressure usually with the point of a reflex hammer.

When the Babinski sign is present, the large toes extends upward and the other toes fan out. The full response is also accompanied by dorsiflexion of the ankle (movement of the toes toward the shin) and flexion of the hip and knee joint. In addition, there may even be a slight contraction or an abduction of the thigh, leading to withdrawal of the leg.

The spinal cord segments involved in the reflex arc being activated are Lumbar 4 and 5 and Sacral 1 and 2.

The Babinski reflex assists in development of joint rotation, especially in the feet, ankles, knees, and hips. It also helps develop muscle tone in the lower part of the body and supports overall freedom of movement. It helps to develop gross motor coordination, which in turn, prepares the child for crawling, standing, walking, and running.

Because of its connection to the vestibular system, it plays an important role in the development of balance, coordination, speech development, and higher-level cognitive skills.

When it fails to integrate, the abnormal response is sometimes referred to as the "Babinski sign". A retained Babinski reflex is often the first (and sometimes only) indication of a serious neurological disease. Medical professionals assess the Babinski reflex to help identify lesions or other damage in the spinal cord and brain. When the reflex is active after age two, it may indicate disorders of the spine or brain such as cerebral palsy. In a baby, the Babinski sign occurs because the corticospinal pathways (running from cerebral cortex down the spinal cord) are not yet fully myelinated. Slow, prolonged contraction of toe extensors may indicate front lobe lesions. Remember in adults, only asymmetry is truly pathological, as is the case with muscle stretch reflexes[cxxxiii].

The Babinski sign can also indicate an abnormality in the motor control pathways leading from the cerebral cortex, and poor gross motor skills such as abnormal gait may be evident. Abnormal gait is characterized by hip rotation, shuffling, or walking on the inside or outside of the feet (leading to excessive wear on these areas of the shoes sole. There may also be dorsiflexion of the toes (toes pointing toward the shin) as well as contraction of the thigh and leg muscles. Running, as well as walking quickly, may be difficult. Ankles may be loose and easily sprained, and cramps may occur in the feet and legs. Furthermore, the individual may have difficulty wearing shoes.

A retained Babinski response can cause a delay in the development of the vestibular system, leading to issues with balance and stability when moving. As a result, a child with a retained Babinski reflex may have delayed or decreased ability to develop higher-level cognition skills such as speech and abstract thinking.

Later in life, we can see the Babinski sign re-emerge in neuropathological conditions such as Amyotrophic lateral sclerosis (ALS), brain tumours, multiple sclerosis, meningitis, Parkinson's, and some forms of polio. Concussions and head injuries, as well as spinal cord injuries, spinal cord tumours, stroke, and spinal tuberculosis can also demonstrate the Babinski sign. It may also appear briefly after a seizure, a marathon, or long walk, or in conjunction with the use of alcohol and drugs.

To summarise, the Babinski reflex emerges about one week after birth. It helps to develop lower body functions such as muscle tone and joint rotation in the feet, ankles, knees, and hips. It also helps develop gross motor coordination, preparing the child for crawling, standing, walking, and running. Because of its connection to the vestibular system, it plays an important role in the development of balance, coordination, speech development, and higher-level cognitive skills. Retention of previously mentioned reflexes such as the Moro, and spinal Galant let alone the FPR may interfere with the smooth integration of the Babinski reflex. Integration should occur by one year but may be delayed until year two. When integration does not occur normally, gross motor skills, joint rotation, and brain/cognitive functions may be jeopardised. Conditions associated with a retained Babinski include autism, cerebral palsy, foot problems as an adult (bunions, flat arches, etc.), stroke, and Parkinson's disease.

Asymmetrical Tonic Neck Reflex

The asymmetrical tonic neck reflex (ATNR) starts 13-18 weeks in utero. It is most prominent between 1 and 4 months of age and should disappear by 3 to 9 months after birth[cxxxiv]. The ATNR begins contributing to foetal development and safety by stimulating the baby's kicks in the womb and providing tactile stimulation for both mother and child. The ATNR allows the baby to make small alterations in its body position in the womb, which is thought to contribute to foetal comfort as well as helping pump circulation in the child's body. The ATNR also stimulates homolateral movement (movement of the limbs on the same side) hence the term asymmetrical. These various movements by the foetus help to develop muscle tone. At this point in utero, the ATNR also has a hand in assisting the development of the vestibular system; these movements send signals into the CNS, and activate loop arcs down the vestibular spinal pathway.

Outside the womb, this reflex is significant for posture of the spine and body, eye-hand coordination, and the tone required in activities like sitting, swimming, playing with a ball, etc. This postural tone is influenced by cortical and subcortical structures, including somatic descending brainstem pathways, descending fibre tracts of monoaminergic system pathways, and limbic system[cxxxv].

As the moment of birth becomes imminent, the ATNR switches gears so that it may accompany the birthing process. The spinal Galant reflex and the ATNR contribute to both flexibility and motility of the foetus' movements as the mother's labour begins. This allows the baby to start to emerge from the uterus in rhythm with the mother's contractions and begin heading down the birth canal. The birth process itself develops the ATNR and other reflexes. Sally Goddard Blythe has noted that ATNR not only supports the birth process but is reinforced by it, thus a vaginal delivery should assist with the integration of the ATNR and other reflexes, whereas there is the thought that C-section and forceps deliveries may interfere with emerging reflexes and later, reflex integration, although more research is needed to confirm this[cxxxvi]. This is another reason mechanical intervention in the birth process can contribute to the continuum issues, primitive reflex retention, apart from their capacity to interrupt craniofacial development.

Once the baby is born, the ATNR pivots once again and begins contributing to various aspects of life.

It is part of the rhythmic movement of the babies' limbs driving the neurological pathways to be laid down connecting them to volitional motor control. In the long term it helps the baby to develop motor skills, including rolling over on their stomach and crawling. The reflex also plays a key role in the development of early eye-hand coordination. The new-born's vision allows him to focus approximately seven inches or 18 centimetres in front of the face, though objects may yet appear unclear as focus is still to yoke the eyes together with practice. When the baby turns his head, the ATNR prompts the arm on the same side to extend, inviting the gaze to follow the arm towards the hand, thus eye hand coordination not the other way around.

This allows the baby's visual field to extend to arm's length and teaches the child that the arms are part of the body and other things are not. They then start to see and grasp objects, stimulating further progression of hand-eye coordination. By about four months, the baby has mature focusing ability an eye yoking.

The ATNR can be usually identified during the first three months of life. To elicit the response, one should rotate the head of the infant to one side while he is lying on his back. Typically, the limbs on the same side will extend while those on the opposite side flex. By four months of age, a mature focusing ability should appear, while neck muscles grow stronger, head control improves, visual abilities grow, and the cortex develops.

Around month 5 the infant will begin to roll, Usually from Back to tummy, this action is associated with integration of the ATNR if There has not been enough time spent practising or rolling was skipped, then the ATNR may not integrate and will start to cause a snowballing to poor integration of other follow-on reflexes.

An active ATNR will be. Demonstrated with the hand foot mouth reflex being generated homolaterally not diagonally. The active ATNR will cause the child to be unable to hold their foot effectively as the limb will extend out to the side when the head turns to look at the foot.

If all goes to plan, the ATNR will begin to integrate, and will be complete by the time the child is between six and seven months old. The ATNR is involved with developing the corpus callosum and drives communication between the left and right cerebral hemispheres. The ATNR will help develop the vestibular system and its mechanisms for balance. The ATNR helps develop the wiring from the semi-circular canals of the inner ear that detect head movement, informing the individual if his head is upright or tilted, even when the eyes are closed. Interestingly when this pathway is developed, the eyes counter-roll in the socket even with the lids closed by reflex to keep the image upright on the retina.

Clearly a disruption in this process can throw the entire system into disorder.

A retained ATNR is responsible for many developmental delays or neurological abnormalities in the developing human. These range from difficulties with movement, coordination, vision, and balance, to issues with cognition, learning challenges, and serious joint and bone misalignment including scoliosis. These issues can then create difficulties with higher order tasks, cognition, and development, including but not limited to crawling and later walking, reading, handwriting, sports, and behaviour.

Again, I raise the chicken egg scenario of the oral fascial maldevelopment, which is leading to the issues as mouth breathing and tongue tie discrepancies resemble the issues caused by a retained reflex such as the Moro or the ATNR.

A retained ATNR disrupts the very foundation of the child's development, impairing the fundamental processes of eye tracking, binocular vision, balance, hand-eye coordination, and bilateral movement. The ATNR is noted to be retained in individuals with educational and/or motor challenges and it tends to be the most common primitive reflex retained or possible the easiest assessed for, so more commonly found. Boys are more commonly affected than girls[cxxxvii].

Midline development is the most important structure both neurologically as well as mechanically. All things start in the centre from the lower brainstem and go up and out. One of the earliest noted issues of a retained ATNR is the inability to bring the hand to the midline. Between the ages of six and twelve months, babies explore the world predominantly by their mouth, typically sucking, chewing, or biting any object that fits in the mouth, acquiring information about texture and shape, flavour if any, and function. Indeed, you could consider the baby's first exploratory tool the mouth more than the eyes and significantly more than the not well controlled hands. However, this behaviour requires the natural integration of the ATNR, allowing the baby to bring the hand to the midline even when his head is turned, it also requires that the oral tissue, the tongue and lips, the fascia to be normal in function and mobility. If there is tethering, the ability to explore will be greatly diminished, which in turn will decrease the neurological return to the brain and may increase oral hypersensitivity and defensiveness with oral use. With the ATNR retained and the ability to bring his hand to the midline impaired, the infant is less able to reach for and put objects into the mouth. Later in life, this midline-crossing challenge can impact the ease of reading, writing, and motor coordination when playing certain sports.

The baby with a retained ATNR can struggle with poor motor coordination and balance, making crawling and logically later on walking difficult. Developmentally we can see difficulty with spatial orientation. This is seen by them struggling to distinguish right from his left. They may also show mixed laterality which is difficulty in choosing a dominant hand, leg, or ear, this is an unconscious activity driven by the CNS not a conscious choice.

Since the child hasn't developed a "dominant" side, there may be a slight hesitancy in their movements, as there is a constant need to decide which side or limb of the body to use to perform a certain task. This creates clumsiness in body movements and confusion or slowing in cognitive thought. In addition, when these processes fail to function automatically, fatigue and overload can occur, which can cause release signs. The child's awkward movements and poor hand-eye coordination can make them appear to be "different" and render them a target for bullying.

The ATNR is highly involved with visual development, when retained, significant impacts may be seen in both vision and reading skills. Over 50 percent and in some places quoted as 95% of children with a retained ATNR are reported to have dyslexia[cxxxviii]. A paper by McPhilips and Jordan-Black suggested that "for many children in mainstream schooling, the attainment of core educational skills may be affected by the persistence of a brainstem mediated reflex system that should have been inhibited in the first year after birth"[cxxxix], these being the ATNR/STNR, the Moro and other reflexes that affect the vestibular-ocular colic systems integration. Harald Blomberg reported that children with dyslexia who received motor exercises and rhythmic movements to integrate the ATNR significantly improved their reading ability compared with a control group[cxl].

As mentioned earlier, the difficulty crossing the midline often experienced when the reflex is retained is one of the factors in dyslexia. Challenges may occur in connection with eye movements, known as tracking or "ocular pursuit". These actions require fixation on an object and moving the eyes in sync with the object's movement in time. They are tiring and cost a lot of energy and concentration. The child's eyes may also not be able to make accurate reflexogenic rapid movements called saccades that are necessary for reading[cxli], losing the space on the line, missing words, or taking too long to complete the task. Saccades are fast sudden shifting of fixation from one target directly to another with precision, think of these actions as being necessary to read along a line hopping from one word to another. Clearly these dysfunctions can lead to comprehension issues as well as spelling and grammar difficulties. The student may find that they are unable to read small print and do better with magnification, only showing the issues as they graduate to books for older children. From large print widely spaced children's versions.

The ATNR helps set the visual distance of the hand in space from the head, but the integration of the reflex helps allow clear vision beyond arm length, thus retention of the ATNR may prevent the development of long-distance vision as well as binocular vision. This difficulty leads to blurring and double images, often causing the child to rub his eyes, and making them red. Some children experience erratic eye movements that make the print appear to jump around. In some cases, they may omit letters, words, or even whole lines when reading, or they may start words or sentences at the end. As the process of reading becomes more difficult, reading comprehension is affected because of this physical strain. The extra effort and intense concentration translates to slower reading, which may in itself also decrease comprehension[cxlii].

Not surprisingly, a retained ATNR is also strongly associated with hand-writing difficulties. When a child turns his head to look at the page, the active ATNR will automatically cause the arm to extend and then cause the fingers to open. Using a pen or pencil will require more effort for the student, and he may compensate by using excessive pressure[cxliii] this can be seen with stabbing and tearing of the paper if using a pen or breaking of a pencil tip regularly. All of this requires intense concentration that occurs at the expense of cognitive processing. As in the case of struggling readers, children with a retained ATNR will find themselves fighting against an "unseen force," namely themselves. Handwriting will suffer in terms of quality and quantity. An overly tight grip can cause cramping and fatigue to set in rapidly, especially in the arm and hand. The frequent "shaking out" of cramped hands is often an indicator of an active ATNR.

A student with active ATNR may have to straighten their arm when writing unable to bend the elbow, to compensate for this awkward posture they may lean back in a chair allowing arm is straight while continuing to write, twisting their body in the seat, or rotating the page to a ninety-degree angle to allow for the outstretched arm. With it difficult for the eyes and hands to cross the midline, in the ATNR child, we can see writing style may be very slanted on the page. These writing difficulties are all under the title dysgraphia.

Some students may read well but be evaluated as lazy or underachieving as the Retained ATNR can make dysgraphia leading to remarks on the report card, must try harder. A retained ATNR can also cause dyscalculia (math difficulties), and manifest as confusion between tens and ones as well as sequencing difficulty.

The retained ATNR does not only affect the child scholastically, but shows up as disturbed sports performance, such as running, bike riding, or rollerblading. Having poor midline capacity, generally lower tone, and poor coordination and an active ATNR tends to make complex actions involving limbs on both sides of the body more difficult to learn.

The brain map has not separated the head from neck or the trunk, therefore when the child tries to move the arm/shoulder the neck muscles or trunk muscles activate at the same time. The children will often perform sports in a clumsy fashion. Swimming which is a school requisite in Australian schools can be a particular challenge due to shoulder restriction. The child may exhibit a splashy rolling style when doing the crawl stroke and as a result, shoulder injuries may develop, they may appear wiggly in the middle, as trunk stabilisation does not occur.

As expected, integration of the ATNR can allow shoulder muscles to relax as the map is better developed and the child can coordinate allowing independent movement of the neck removing unnecessary structural stress upon joints and allowing normal muscle function.

Cortical map smudging is where there is not discrete localisation of motor sensory neuronal pools relating to body parts such as the head, shoulder, and arms, this can at least partially be caused by a retained ATNR. This smudging stops the brain activating discrete precise movements and as such can sometimes make the fingers open, and hold objects drop when straightening the arm. This generates difficulty for the child in manipulating objects such as forks or spoons; especially if the visual field is activated at the table by other people causing the head to turn; these children are often considered a "messy eater". Imagine the difficulty for the ATNR child learning to ride a bicycle. The child will lose their balance when movement of the head to the left or right causes the arm and leg to automatically straighten in the same direction., notwithstanding the vestibular issues and the trunk not stabilising over the pelvis properly. They will likely have many grazes and scars especially on the lower limbs, and not enjoy this form of activity.

Another difficulty associated with the active ATNR is that it can interact with neck proprioceptors and a retained tonic labyrinthine reflex creating an antagonistic effect on the neck and spine[cxliv] joints and muscles. The antagonistic actions of the labyrinth reflex for the head tilt or rotation are opposed by the neck reflexes causing upright trunk posture and stabilising action to extremities acting as a single system to joint and bone misalignment, including curvature of the spine leading to scoliosis[cxlv]. Keith Keen conducted a study that demonstrated a link between the retained ATNR and scoliosis in school children, concluding that ATNR testing may be useful in early scoliosis identification. This is especially interesting when we pair the consideration with our zebrafish studies which found that alteration in the level of nutrition and the flow of CSF in the developing foetus led to a long-term scoliosis outcome in the offspring.

It seems like there is no separation between what is cause and effect, as they all develop together.

The primitive reflexes all give service for a period of time before they should integrate and then become postural reflexes, which aid the next step in the child's development. If the normal integration does not occur and a reflex is retained, abnormal movement patterns can occur unconsciously and need to be actively controlled by brain power. Think of a child with a retained Asymmetrical Tonic Neck Reflex (ATNR), they turn the head to the left and the back may arch, and the Left arm and or leg extends forward.

This might also look like a constantly tight upper trapezius and neck shoulder muscles in an adult person, more on one side. The constant need to control the involuntary muscle movements using conscious thought requires a lot of extra energy to be diverted from normal processes such as learning, growing, thriving, to suppressing the twitch. This leads to fatigue in the child and potentially emotional lability. The scenario makes it even harder to maintain a normal development trajectory. What can then occur is the brain will continue to try to develop around the "stuck" spot in the brain stem, the cerebrum tries to develop normally, but there is a lack of full spectrum information coming through. The pathways from the periphery can be slow or unclear and the processing of the information can be garbled, leading to developmental dysfunction in the higher cortical functions, and movement pattern development of the body. This can be seen as difficulty expressing or interpreting facial emotions, greater vigilance and startle response or jerky stilted body movement patterns, amongst many others.

It is important for the maturation process that the child is placed on its belly a lot, so the muscles in the back and abdomen have plenty of exercise and activation. By 6 weeks a paediatric trained practitioner should be able to see if head control is appropriately developed, children who have been placed on their back a lot will not have developed these neck control muscles effectively through a lack of movement opportunity, think spending lots of time in car seats. If we cast our mind back to the previous section, we remember that issues with tongue/oral eye up activation early after birth can alter head muscle control mirroring the ATNR issues and is also associated with the retained FPR/Moro response. This could be seen as the beginning of the obstacles to reflex integration, considering the baby develops its body control from brain down and middle out pattern. Brain stem, to cerebellum, via the spinocerebellar tracts, up to the cortex, down to the body to develop neurological control loops.

The Landau Reflex

The landau reflex is an interesting reflex as it starts later than most of the others and integrates much later than the other reflexes. It is imperative for it to integrate as we will discuss, as it is associated with the capacity to experience joy, thus maladaptation of this reflex may cause mood issues and dysphoria in later life.

Its significant feature is that it interplays with other reflexes to aid in body development. The trigger for the Landau reflex is elicited when the baby is held flat under the stomach and is lifted up, like playing aeroplane, the baby should lift their head and extend the trunk and legs, they should laugh and smile. This reflex is seen as an expression of joy and happiness and is associated with the "affect" of play[cxlvi]. If this is not integrated the adult may have difficulty experiencing joy or happiness later in life. According to research by Mitchell "The Landau reflex is present if the infant raises his head and arches their back with the concavity upwards"[cxlvii].

As noted the Landau reflex starts after birth, it should first appear at three months of age and will lose its usefulness, to integrate by about three years.

It is considered normal to activate the reflex in infants from the age of about 3 months onwards and it should become increasingly difficult to evoke after the age of one year, while not out of the question to be present to some degree at 3, the absence of the response in infants over the age of 3 months is associated with motor weakness issues such as in cerebral palsy, motor neurone disease and mental retardation thus its importance as an indicator of normal development.

The Landau reflex combines neurological aspects of labyrinthine, neck and visual reactions and therefore will be essential for development of position sense and location of head, neck and body in space in response to gravity. It has been described as a "righting reaction", in which the body responds optimally to gravity.

The Landau reflex contributes to development in several important ways, including helping coordinate head neck vestibular position that allows binaural hearing, meaning that both ears work together to allow location of a sound source in relation to the body, a 3-dimensional sonar locator if you will. As you'd expect the landau reflex promotes the development of vestibular-ocular position integration allowing the ability to distinguish horizontal and vertical lines and the capacity for three-dimensional vision, depth perception, as well as tracking of objects and ultimately the capacity to calculate an object's speed in relation to the head. This is critical for survival; it allows the brain to make defence decisions and determine strategy to avoid injury.

The reflex also contributes to the development of posture and muscle tone. By helping to coordinate the upper and lower parts of the body – including the ability to lift the head and chest and maintain postural control – the child is supported as he learns to stand and then walk. The capacity for head righting is a hallmark of this reflex, as is the muscle tone required for extension from the neck down through the core, legs, and feet.

Conversely, if the reflex has not appeared by the age of six months, it may indicate the presence of neurological damage, including cerebral palsy. And is a reason for a medical assessment. From the point of view of my thesis the landau reflex appears incredibly important.

As we have discussed, if the child does not develop appropriate head position control, then the system compensates by activating anterior cervical muscles to hold the head up and the airway open. Anterior head carriage must be compensated for at the other end of the chain by retroversion of the pelvis and increased tension to the iliacus and psoas muscles. This alteration in postural position will make it harder to activate a typical landau reflex. The question then becomes is it alteration to the neural circuits that regulate landau activation that drives this postural change or does something else drive change in postural cues, leading to maldevelopment of the landau reflex. Sadly, there is no answer in the current literature.

The Landau reflex integrates with other neural reflexes which helps develop the child into a functional adult. The tonic labyrinthine reflex (TLR) and symmetrical tonic neck reflex (STNR) combine neurologically with the landau reflex allowing gravity fed head righting, which becomes body position in space, up and down, left, and right coordinate locomotion as well as knowledge of where our body begins and ends. However, if the reflex does not integrate appropriately, we can see problems with body movement, cognitive development, as well as mood and behaviour, making it difficult in the educational environment. Schools are not forgiving places either in the playground or the curriculum for kids with a difference or two, that don't take in information in the neurotypical manner or behave quite like the others.

Children with a disintegrated landau may appear stiff with lower-body awkwardness and have issues with head righting, keeping it upright in response to gravity, not squished down and forward. The shoulders and upper body may be flexed, with increased anterior head carriage. The limb joints such as the knee or elbow may seem to be locked, making it difficult to bend the body forward or to adjust muscle tone in rapidly changing movements such as hopping, jumping, and skipping. This is due to competing neural pathways firing when they shouldn't be on both sides of the joint[cxlviii]. This is joint muscle antagonism.

From the emotive difficulty perspective children and adults may exhibit difficulty with many aspects of life. Not being assertive, nor responding to danger appropriately, difficulty transitioning from activities to another focus. Teenagers and adults whose Landau reflex remain unintegrated may display procrastination, with a strong avoidance drive, their sense the movement of time can be off leading to habitual lateness for appointments, the breaking of commitments and poor social connection.

As I noted, the school yard is an unforgiving place and once the child enters school, a retained Landau reflex can play havoc. To start with the avoidance behaviour, procrastination, and inability to maintain time sequence to keep appointments means getting to school on time is a nightmare, not to mention difficulty with task swapping, as well as an inability to concentrate on details or process new information, makes the retention of learning a major challenge, students may also display poor organisational skills and have difficulty completing work to hand in on time.

Dr. Thomas Hanna has been studying the primitive reflexes and their effect on the somatic body since before I was born, setting up education and research facilities to enhance the understanding of the mind body connection.

Dr Hanna has referred to the Landau reflex as the "Joy Reflex" referring to the infant's joyful exploration of the world with his expanding movement[cxlix]. This makes some sense as the joy hit re-enforces the behaviour, the spine head extension , allows the ability to view the world an starts the ability to move in the world, without the Landau, the ability to start crawling which allows cross crawl patterns (CER) to lead to walking is restricted, therefore reenforcing this pattern is essential for survival, which I believe is why the action is co-activated with a strong chemical soup inducing joy, to keep it happening. I would have you consider that a lack of appropriate movement in any age of development has negative consequences to the end outcome of the human. Restriction is often unhelpful, including ankyloglossia.

Dr Hanna further links inappropriate muscle contraction due to a retained landau as being associated with the spinal pain of people over 40 (continuing my thoughts about movement restriction being negative), suggesting that about 80 percent of those in the business community with spinal pain, will result from a chronically contracted spine caused by the unintegrated Landau reflex.

The Retained landau child may exhibit self-denial, by not asking for what they need nor accepting kindness when it is offered. This condition can also pave the way for depression or a lack of emotions.

Joy is what happens to us when we are able to realise how wonderful life is once the Landau reflex is integrated. Notably, a person who is depressed can have difficulty replicating and activating their body into the Landau position.

Integration of the Landau can help to relieve depression, strengthen concentration, and focus, and improve posture and muscle tone. The Landau plays an integral part of our development, bringing feelings of peace and happiness.

There is so much that the Landau touches and it being retained or poorly integrated or released after chemical/physical brain trauma can create havoc for the adult.

In addition, there are several associated conditions with the Landau reflex including ADHD, autism, cerebral palsy, depression, and Down's syndrome, that if seen the reflex should be assessed and activities instigated to inhibit the reflex.

Symmetrical Tonic Neck Reflex (STNR)

This is another interesting reflex, that similar to the Landau is not apparent at birth and comes into play later on, occasionally the Symmetrical Tonic Neck Reflex (STNR) is active very briefly just after birth to assist the infant in pushing itself up on Mum in the process of finding her breast) The STNR could be considered a postural reflex or at least part of the transition to them. It appears at six to nine months of age and should integrate quickly (hence its transitional nature), generally between nine and eleven months of age, along with the ATNR. However according to Bruin, the ATNR and STNR can be found in children up to 9 years of age[cl]. Bruin further suggested that these reflexes may still be involved in motor control in these children, whereas I suggest that it's an abnormal motor neural pattern and therefore the use of this circuit is a compensation and inappropriate for development at any age past one year.

The STNR is considered to be a transitory reflex assisting the child's brain in the development of the tonic labyrinthine reflex circuitry to control head on neck movements, head righting, visual targeting and biaural location. There is a possibility that the STNR is simply a stage in the development of the tonic labyrinthine reflex and not a true reflex of its own, in the "extension" form which may make Bruin's assertions of children having it available for use at 9 years old more palatable but suggesting that the TLR is the culprit that has not integrated fully.

The STNR is involved in the process of visual accommodation with co-ordination with other reflexes including the ATNR. Accommodation is the process of moving the eyes from a far object to a focus point on a near object closer to the face. In the infant this is useful to see an object away from the body, such as mum bringing a spoon of food towards the infant's mouth, the baby watches the hand all the way in. This process is object tracking which activates visual fixation and visual pursuit. Accommodation can also be seen when the infant has an item that perhaps they should not have, they hold the object in front of their face, look at it, to their parent's face, then back to the object before stuffing it in their mouth.

The ATNR causes the arm to extend as the head turns, with the eye following the hand, the STNR aids visual development from near too far as well as visual horizon stabilisation to draw the hand towards the face, a tango of reflexes working together. This is seen (no pun intended) as the baby rocks back and forward on hands and knees. As the head rises, far vision is activated, and the reverse occurs as the head lowers (near vision is activated), both actions activate the TLR and the entrainment of the eyes to the horizon. These reflexes are essential to yoke the eye movements together. Most people reading this book take for granted that their eyes are paired and moved together to give depth perceptions, however binocular vision, is not immediate after birth and the muscle control and neural circuits that create this essential sensory perception is another practiced capacity created by STNR's contributions combined with the other reflexes (ATNR, TLR). The STNR also helps create hearing lateralisation and biaural (hearing) sound location for sound sensory perception.

To some degree, what the STNR influences is not surprising, "Symmetrical" is the key word. Both eyes, both ears, and both sides of the body. The STNR helps integrate and co-ordinate the bilateral and top and bottom movement patterns of the body such as in crawling, it's a cross crawl pattern using opposite arm to leg moving together, while stabilising the trunk/abdomen and maintain neck tone in a head up forward position. This indicates that the STNR reaches up across the corpus collosum to create the descending motor pathways and the feedback loops that start as a reflex and become active conscious movement, then become unconscious imprinted motor patterns. This is seen in action that you don't have to think about each foot fall and arm swing when running or climbing a set of stairs, you just tell the brain run and go.

The STNR can be seen as essential for tool use, the first major even is co-ordination of upper body extension while on knees as part of crawling, (this also includes intervention from the landau reflex), head up gravity fed, which allow the hands to be free to manipulate objects. From here, the baby will continue to defy gravity leading to enough central tone and head control to drive towards standing.

The normal demonstration of the STNR reflex is seen in the infant when the baby raises her head and extends the spine, then their arms straighten, the legs bend, and the buttocks lower onto the ankles. In counterpoint, when the baby lowers their head, the arms bend, and the legs try to straighten. This can be demonstrated in adults with a retained STNR when on hands and knees. Eyes closed, we passively flex the head, the elbows might bend, and when the head/neck is extended the hips and knees flex, buckling the bottom towards the feet.

By month six Crawling preparation movements start. Issues with the STNR reflex integration and progression will interfere with coordinated movements in crawling, the long-term consequences of skipping crawling and having an active STNR is seen with a lack of motivation to apply themselves and issues with transitions to new things, pulling back. An active STNR reflex, will be seen in the 6-month-old infant as legs being stretch as soon as the head lifts to orientate to view them.

If only a single step in the child's motor development is skipped or not practised enough, alteration in pathway myelination between the cerebellum, brainstem, and cortex, with the outcome being retained primitive reflexes and consequences showing up in later life.

What does a retained STNR look like? In infancy, the baby may not be able to coordinate their upper and lower body as needed to crawl on hands and knees; instead, she might "bear walk" on her hands and feet or bum shuffle on a hip/thigh pulling themselves along and may not hit the usual 12-month milestone of standing to start the process of walking upright.

The retained STNR leaves the infant who is trying to crawl, with a risk of arm collapse as the head rocks (Infront of the centre of gravity) forward, to combat this the infant may have to extend her head upward, which alters eye horizon regulation and is behind the centre of gravity to enable bearing weight on the forearms for crawling. Now let's go back to a concept we discussed before in the discussion of the ATNR. If the child does not activate appropriate head position control due to the ATNR not integrating appropriately leading to weak midline neck muscles, the compensation is to recruit more muscles to hold the head up, this causes an anterior movement of head upon neck, which also causes hyperactivation of the suboccipital muscles, which as we can see from the STNR will cause and alteration of the eye position and accommodation control and possibly alteration of yoking. The upper body alteration creates a compensatory activation of lower body flexion including iliopsoas muscles, the hamstrings and a postural alteration in the pelvic position, the consequence of which includes inflexibility in the lower body, greater difficulty maintaining postural tone to support body weight on arms and legs for crawling, and possibly developmental delay of future milestones. Activation of the appropriate body reflexes allows the infant to increase muscle strength development which feeds the brain and strengthens motor pathways to become unconscious motor control.

Thus, the more "normal " accurate crawling activity is performed, the better the child becomes at it leading to brain development and more body tone. As you can imagine poor control of the head due to STNR/ATNR retention will lead to less muscle use and tone development, leading to low tone of both midline structures and peripheral muscles. This hypotonicity further aggravates the ability to maintain stance when trying to stand and or walk. It will display as balance disorders and increased flexor tone in the neck shoulders and pelvis seen as a stooped posture, flexed hips and bent knees. In the adult this is rounded shoulders, a buffalo or dowager's hump or slumped low back or sway back. They have a tendency towards an increase in tendon irritation and joint pain, low back pain, neck pain headaches and TMJ pain. While all of these physical changes occur, they will usually have poor airway control and will often suffer mouth breathing, the consequence of which is increased a shift in blood acidity, oxidative stress, calcium release into the tissue, creating soft tissue tension pain and symptom creation purely due to mouth breathing. So, let's take a second to consider the last paragraph in relation to tongue tie and oral maldevelopment syndrome- the Continuum. All of the same dysfunctions occur and can be laid at the feet of oral fascial tethering, pulling the head forward, changing the eye position in the head, how we use the spine and compensatory action of the neuromuscular development. Human development is hard wired to continue even when not perfect so the compensations become " normal" for the child, we may call these retained primitive reflexes or we may call it oral facial dysfunction but they occur contiguously with one another, and both physical interventional and neurophysiological rehabilitation needs to occur to drive the child back to a normal trajectory. We take development too much for granted that it just "occurs" and is always perfect.

By this stage I am hoping you can see that the essential nature of primitive and postural reflexes for human development and their critical importance too midline structure development both postural as well as the neuro-cortical loops that help develop eye control, respiratory rhythm, stress, and vigilance response all of which contribute to mouth breathing, sleep regulation and general human health. Ultimately this section is to help the reader learn about neural pathways that are essential for functional development of the child which drives the form of our structure. These reflexes are commonly glossed over by neuroscience and medicine in favour of big brain control and importance as if how we get there is almost instantaneous or unimportant. As you should also now be aware the retention of these reflexes is associated or possibly causative of many pathological conditions including ADHD, autism spectrum disorders, OCD, anxiety and many others.

Further I wanted you to consider that the retention of primitive reflexes, leads to compensation, the creation of a "get around", a "Skyhook" which we call non-neurotypical development, and this may actually underlie diseases of the mature adult. I wish for you to understand that they (the primitive reflexes not integrated) contribute to the continuum of human health and disease, that any patients that attend their physician for depression, generalised anxiety, ADHD, Parkinson's disease etc, should be assessed for retention of primitive reflexes. We should perhaps not consider their symptoms as frontal release signs, but more that the reflexes never integrated and are now showing up as problems that the patient can no longer functionally compensate for, and have become annoying enough to seek help with or a diagnosis of.

Further that all of these reflexes are associated with airway issues and sleep fragmentation since early childhood (technically 5 weeks in utero), as the **FPR** and the midline mouth structures including oral fascia's and the cartilaginous cells for facial structure both develop at this point – together. It is currently impossible to separate their occurrences from one another, thus the maldevelopment of one is likely associated with or causative of maldevelopment of the other.

8

Muscle Development and Primitive Reflexes

It's important to remember long-term that alteration in muscle control development patterns can lead to hypertonic and hypotonic cervical muscles in the neck and throat and top of chest/back, along with difficulty holding the weight of the head. This can lead to recruitment of other muscles to help hold the head weight up and can lead to issues with airway patency during sleep.

Muscle recruitment patterns may not be obvious and may be at the other end of the chain.

The skeletal spine in its brilliance has balanced motor units, including both bones as well as the muscles surrounding each joint. One above to balance one below. In the spine this reciprocal relationship is call the Lovett Brother relationship. From a paper by Charles Blum "The spine appears to function with a specific harmonious movement as an individual walks, runs, and otherwise performs daily activities. The vertebra working in conjunction with each other, such as the 1st lumbar and 5th cervical, are known as Lovett Brothers"[cli] , these are pair motor units and are used by the brain to maintain upright posture with the centre of gravity balance to allow the most efficient locomotion. The muscles of the spine and trunk therefore have to be recruited to maintain the head over the pelvis, if the muscles of the neck are well and adaptive recruitment occurs, then a position of the neck which may be anterior to the centre of gravity, will cause the body to recruit automatic balancing muscle in the low back and pelvis to reposition the lower body under the head and maintain posture. Consider that this is part of the purpose of the primitive reflexes such as the Landau, the TLR, STNR and ATNR, they automated muscle recruitment patterns to maintain efficient locomotion as an adult.

Long term if this postural disfunction becomes entrained with inappropriate head position and poor upper muscle balance, then hip muscles will stay contracted, to manage gravity. They will become shorter and tighter, never feeling relaxed, as they will constantly be recruited to maintain posture. This will lead to a loss of hip and low back position and mobility.

The Temporomandibular joint and the SI joint are reciprocal pairs according to SOT research from Dr De Janette and others[cliii], therefore the facial dysmorphia which causes narrow palate and mandible growth change, will alter the TMJ and dentition, often leading to airway distress and orthodontics as previously discussed, however this reciprocity may also lead to structural change in the lumbo-pelvic bones and motor pairs. This can be seen in shorter mouth opening, as well as tight hamstrings, calves and psoas muscles, and an inability to bend, squat or touch the toes.

Posture and fascia

Let's consider posture a bit further. This again is a concept that is commonly taken for granted, it is considered an issue of laziness or poor focus by the body owner if posture is not good. We consider it a response to bad habits or work activity, we blame mobile device use and a number of external influences but never consider that this may be an internal issue, reflexogenic, respiratory driven or fascial in nature.

Fascia as a definition: The Fascia is made up of sheets of connective tissue that is found below the subcutaneously[cliii].

Tissues like this hold things together, separate muscles, keep blood vessels open, surround organs, and so on. Surgeons have historically been the primary users of the term fascia to refer to the dissectible tissue surrounding the body's internal organs, muscles, and bones. The term has recently been expanded to encompass cells that form and maintain the extracellular matrix, as well as all soft tissues in the body that are based on collagen. The revised definition now includes certain tendons, ligaments, bursae, endomysium, perimysium, and epimysium. Fascia is used by the body to entrain position to use the least amount of muscle energy, this includes when asleep. The importance of this is that the fascia if over tight and short will pull on the neck and chest, it can alter the hip position.

Fascia is unlike muscle; it is only one directional and cannot be commanded to relax by the brain. It resists longitudinal stretch, and will force the skeleton to move itself to decrease tension in the tissue, to reduce pain and tissue discomfort. To maintain upright posture when fascia is mechanical short due to growth disruption requires constant activity stretch and release or surgical intervention to reduce the tension upon the spine and midline structures, thus one of the reasons to do the Tongue tie surgeries. The issue being that as soon as conscious drive to maintain upright posture wains, either due to fatigue, focus on another object that is not posture or unconsciousness, such as when asleep the tension returns to the fascia and posture will correct itself to what is considered a flexor position, as this follows the line of ease in the skeletal structure, moves the tongue out of the airway and is in keeping with most of our activities of daily living.

All these activities, reading, computers, driving etc, have the body curving forward.

As you can see in the following the image fascia is a top to bottom connective tissue. It starts in the mouth surrounding the tongue and goes down the throat and neck, through the diaphragm, into the hips down the legs to the tip of the big toe in one long connective tension fibrous strip.

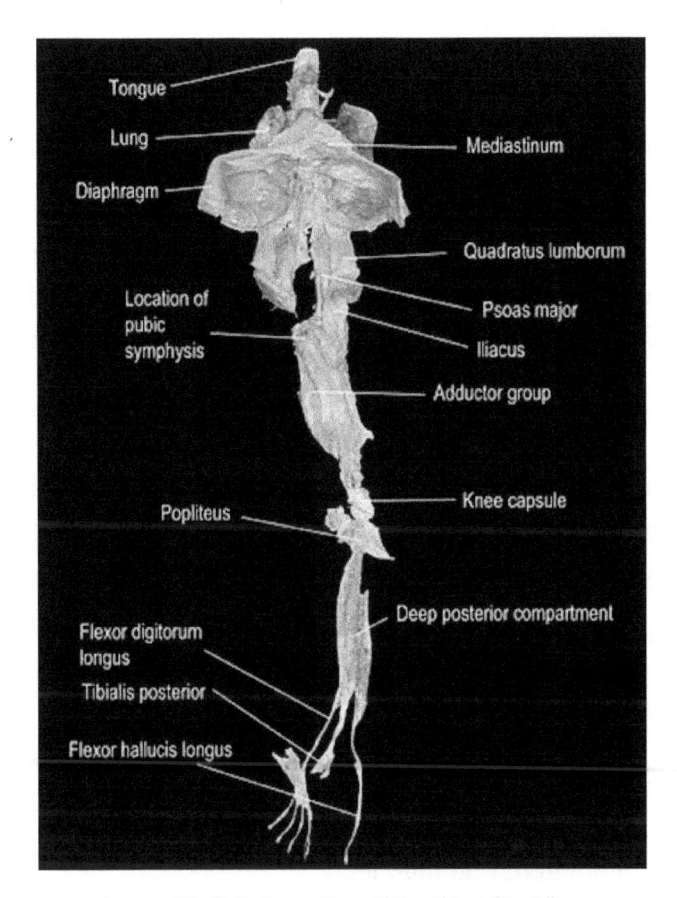

Image 25. Full dissection of the deep front line fascia from tongue tip to the tip of the big toe. Note this is one long piece of connective tissue. From seminar hand out but also seen https://basicmedicalkey.com/the-deep-front-line/

Accessory muscles and posture

This tension is further aggravated by breathing patterns. Stressed breathing or fatigued breathing or poor learned pattern from mouth breathing, where the cycle shortens and quickens, uses less diaphragm drive and more accessory muscle involvement.

When extra power is required, as in exercise or by those with airway pathologies like COPD, the accessory muscles of respiration (muscles in the trunk other than the diaphragm) help out[cliv].

The diaphragm is the primary muscle involved in inspiration during normal calm breathing, with support from the abdominal and external intercostal muscles. Whereas inspiration is an active process, expiration is passive due to the elastic recoil of the rib cage and related components[clv].

However, the accessory muscles are also activated in times of stress and during postural disadvantage, such as shoulder rounding, airway obstruction, and head forwards posturing.

The accessory respiratory muscle groups include:

Accessory inspiratory muscles

- Sternocleidomastoid muscles
- Scalene muscles – Anterior, middle, and posterior
- External intercostal muscles
- Pectoralis major
- Pectoralis minor
- Serratus anterior
- Latissimus dorsi
- Serratus posterior superior

Accessory expiratory muscles

- Abdominal muscles
- Internal intercostal muscles

The accessory muscles are all covered in fascia as is the diaphragm. They are supported by these connective tissues when fatigued, however this can lead to sensations of tension and discomfort that may not be relieved with rest, stretching or activities such as massage.

The muscles of the chest neck and back will become conditioned over time to hold posture to maintain airway, as respiratory drive is one of if not the most motivators of human behaviour, the brain will drive posturing to make the airway function open and efficient even at the expense of other areas that the educated mind might consider equally important.

This is why postural change is not due to laziness nor primarily driven by our activities of daily action such as device use driving or holding a book to read. There are much deep drivers at play that must be answered.

In fact, we have been complaining about posture and blaming it on one thing or another for over one hundred years, it's all a continuum of changing the narrative to fit the observation, not looking at the reason for the posture to change. I love the juxtaposition of the below picture. It makes a mockery of the current catch cry blaming the mobile device, the phone the tablet laptops and computers. Blaming our current tools is very short sited and doesn't give any consideration to human behaviour or to the purpose behind fascia. If you think about it, most of our activities are down and in front of us, driving, reading a book, giving a massage, making dinner stirring a saucepan, all of these things are anterior and forward body postures that activate anterior chain muscles, and require stabilisation with the posterior chain to maintain balance.

The fascia works to allow the least amount of muscle energy use, to maintain a position that we activate regularly. Fascia has unique properties, including elasticity combine with stiffness, that allow it to resist gravity without requiring the same amount of energy input as a muscle does, it is less tiring on the body.

However, everything has a cost. Tight fascia does not have a great blood supply and does not therefore have great oxygenation, which can lead to oxidative stress, when movement is not abundant to drive fluid through it. If you happen to have midline fascial maldevelopment, i.e. short tense fascia's in the case of tongue tie, then there will be a displacement of force in the anterior and posterior kinetic chains which you can't get away from, leaving the person, with chronic tension in the neck, shoulders and upper back which will be aggravated by long term postural ques such as computer use. This tension is not relieved for any noted length of time by stretching or fascial release techniques, it always comes back as it is literally built in. Patients will often complain of burning pain in the tissue, especially near fascial anchor points, such as the spinous of T6, where the trapezius muscle attaches from head forward sitting posture. Practitioners tend to get hung up on the correlation not the cause. The computer use did not cause the fascial tension, it highlighted it. In my opinion, most of our problems come from unconscious actions and behaviours to enhance survival such as from protecting our airway, including opening it up at night from the risk of oral structure collapse.

First Principles • 189

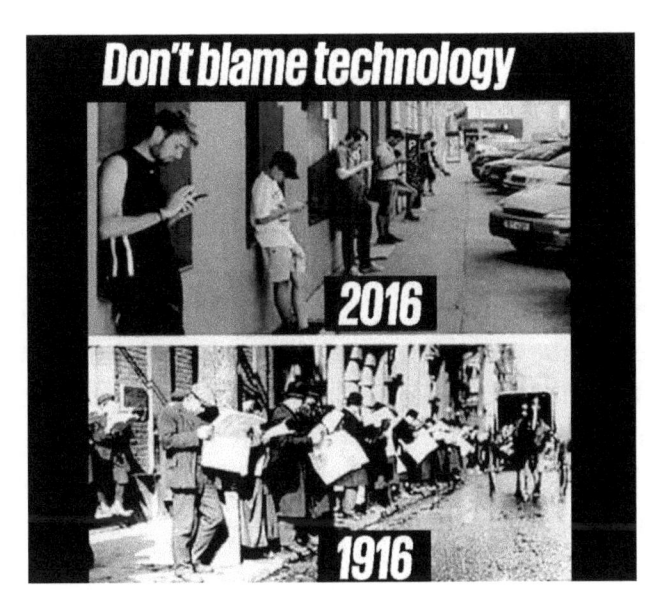

Image 26: Don't blame technology. Demonstrates that hunched forward neck bent posture is nothing new and has been going on for more than 100 years.

THIS IS one of the reasons that tongue tie release can be helpful to long term health and directly to posture. Why interventions that improve airway such as the Myo-nozzle, Myotherapy, orthotropic activity, orthodontics, ENT surgeries and physical and neurological rehabilitation, and cranial chiropractic are imperative to perform and maintain, especially in older patients whose bodies have grown into compensations, away from optimal, bad habits (so to speak) have been encoded into the reflexogenic motor repertoire and will need long term conditioning to learn new better ones, and maintain more optimal posture.

Posture in of itself as noted previously has a series of possible permutations, partially due to the pairing of motor units, structural limitations of the bones, balance actions to stand, the primitive reflexes and the drive to maintain airway to furnish the brain with blood. The pelvis can rotate forward or backwards, either sagging in the middle or pot belly /duck bum posture, while the neck will shift the head to maintain centre of gravity over the hips and feet to allow movement to occur. Competing drives occur at the same time, including, balance, defence- including the ability to see far into the distance, with biaural sound, and the arms free to use tools. All however pale when compared to the strength of the drive to protect and maintain airway. Thus, my proposition that most of our long-term postural deviations (barring from trauma) is really to maintain the airway then is influenced by the other drives in descending order of importance to their value upon survival.

First Principles • 191

WE CAN SEE these patterns in the below photos.

Upright posture:

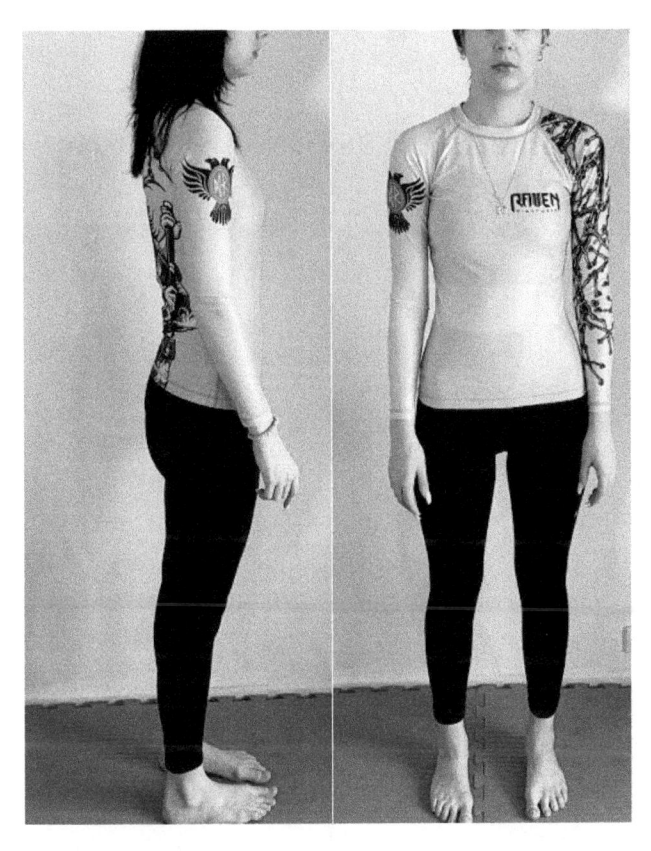

Image 27 and 28: Demonstrate upright from the front and side view. Head is over pelvis, over the feet.

SAGGED in the middle head forward posture with activation of sub occipital muscles.

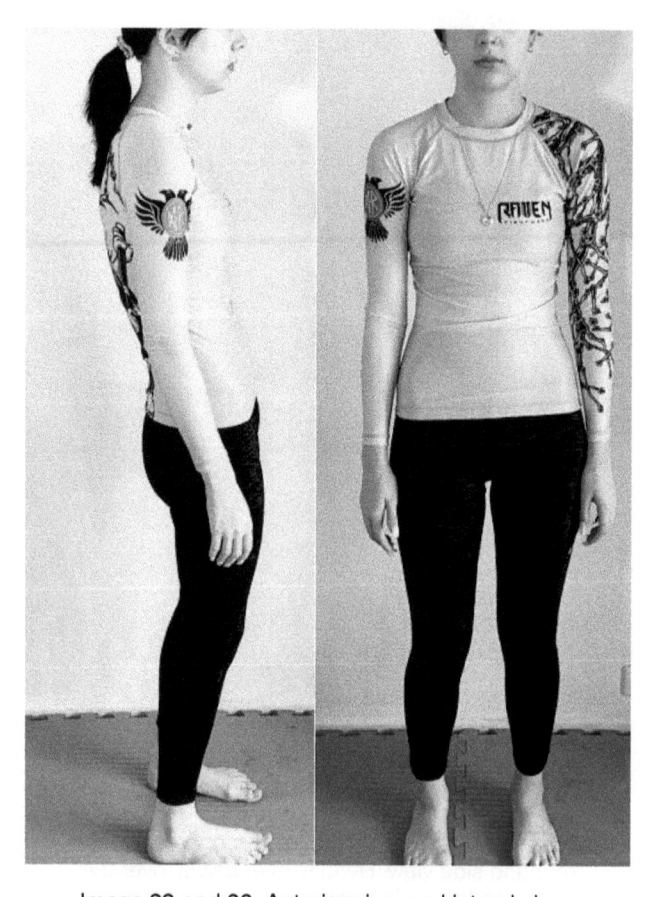

Image 29 and 30: Anterior view and lateral view. Demonstrate Head forward posture with compensatory pelvic tilt, giving a sagged in the middle posture. Note the medial deviation of the knees and the pelvis has gone forward to maintain posture under the head.

CLOSE-UP OF ANTERIOR head and neck with cervical activation, note the tension on the tongue and airway,

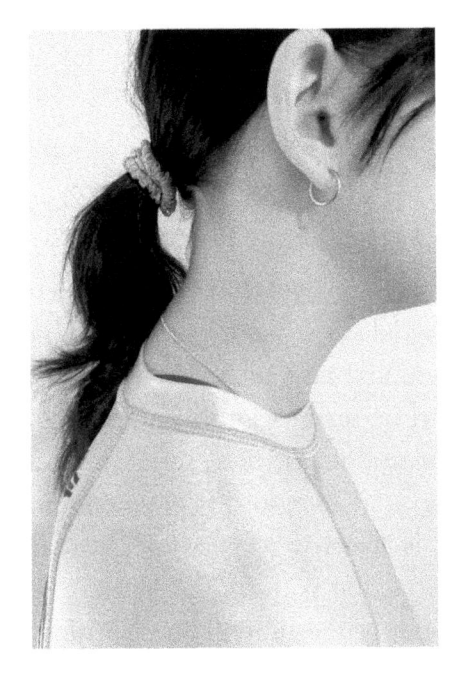

Image 31. Close up of the Anterior view demonstrating head forward posture associated with tight tongue fascia, rounding of the shoulders and elongation and protrusion of the throat.

The role above the brainstem in child development

The main function of the Right hemisphere is gestalt orientated, viewing the combined picture to give an overview. If viewing the word house, the left brain perceives the different letter shapes while the right sees the whole word and gives an appropriate image if understood. Interestingly according to Gilchrist in his seminal book the master and his emissary Iain McGilchrist points out that the hemispheres compete to provide meaning and control the sensory data provided to the cortex[clvi]. The cortex is where consciousness is actuated, it allows planning, and to carryout thought, as well as learn, and move new learnings to store as fixed action patterns in longer term memory.

The cerebellum is primarily responsible for co-ordination of fixed action patterns and learned movements, it is also responsible for modulation of all emotional outputs.

The limbic system is also involved with the short-term memory and emotions and is considered the place where they are stored and activated from, it gives flavour and saliency to the data we process. The amygdala is a major part of the limbic system and regulates the emotional content to an experience. This part of our brain can activate unconsciously and participates in the fight flight flee response and fear. These connections are important as part of learning and long-term potentiation. If an action pattern/emotion is learned when under threat, the amygdala connects the fixed action pattern and layers it with the emotion that was playing out at the time of the learning, such as fear or anxiety, and will be triggered sometimes when the pattern is recalled. This learning, situation, or experience will potentially not store fully as a memory or be associated with negative ones. This can lead to repercussions of an unexpected nature. As with the primitive reflexes that can be activated at inopportune moments unexpectedly, so can learned behaviours that have occurred under stress can be activated by exposure to a stimulus or trigger that reminds the sensorium but not necessarily the cortex of the events that occurred when the learning ensued. This is of course made worse if the primitive reflexes such as the Moro or FPR is inappropriately active in the person.

The lack of integration allows inappropriate ungated ascending signals from the lower brain and brain stem to trigger motor patterns that manifest as either emotion or movement unbidden. This could be part of Tourette's syndrome, but it will leave the person feeling uptight and stressed without reason.

Frontal Release Signs

As the brain matures and develops, areas within the cortex and suspected to be specifically in the frontal lobes exert a descending inhibitory effect on the primitive reflexes that we have discussed above, causing the reflex to "disappear". This is the whole purpose of "integration". In the adult we can observe disease processes disrupting the inhibitory pathway control of the reflexes allowing the reflex to be "released" from inhibition. This means the primitive reflex can be elicited when it shouldn't be, hence the term "frontal release sign". This is noted in diseases such as frontal dementias. However, in some people the reflex may never have fully. Integrated and may have existed since infancy and may be considered a frontal release as against a primitive reflex. This raises the question as to whether retention of the reflex sets one up for pathology, and why we are not looking at these reflexes as a screening tool earlier in life across broad bases of the population.

The six reflexes in commonly considered as frontal release signs when retained, serve as markers or indicators of impairment in the frontal lobes. These six include the hands-grasping, Babkin palmomental, sucking, rooting, glabellar tap, and snout reflexes. These reflexes can be "released," or become active again when frontal lobe damage occurs, or perhaps nerve integrated?

Medicine considers the hands-grasping reflex assessment to be the most useful for detecting frontal lobe damage.

The Sucking Reflex

The sucking reflex emerges in the womb between eighteen and twenty-eight weeks in utero[clvii]. It is present in most preterm and term babies and the sucking reflex will usually integrate between three and four months of age in most normally developing children[clviii]. Along with the rooting reflex, the sucking reflex helps develop mouth movements for eating, keeping in mind function drives form, this means that if there is an alteration to the normal capacity of the sucking reflex, perhaps the tongue does not move easily and firmly in a wave like function to pressure the breast against the hard palette then the consequence is that the Roof of the mouth may not develop the appropriate shape to form the bite, and the floor of the sinuses. This reflex ultimately will help with the development of speech, which clearly will be affected by a maldevelopment of the sucking reflex and the structure of the mouth tongue and other oral structures, or issues with breathing the nasium and airway.

As one would imagine the sucking reflex involves sucking movements by the lips and oral structures including the wave like pressuring of the tongue against the palette, and when is most strongly elicited by stimulus to the palette or when the lips are stroked or touched. Clearly from a survival viewpoint it can be considered one of the most important reflexes as along with the rooting reflex below it is essential for finding and ingesting food. It becomes part of a co-ordinated triad sucking- swallowing- breathing reflex and should be functional by 36 weeks in utero. By the third month, sucking should become a conscious controlled activity, not just a reflex, considering that sucking is a sensation that the infant considers pleasurable and will participate in even when not for nutritive purposes[clix].

The Rooting Reflex

Similar to the sucking reflex, the Rooting Reflex emerges between twenty-four and twenty-eight weeks in utero, definitely by 35 weeks[clx] and is as noted essential for infant survival due to the ability to find food. If all goes to plan it will integrate at three to four months after birth again similar to its mate, the sucking reflex. We elicit this reflex by lightly touching the cheek area near the nasal fold, or a light touch can be applied around the outside edge of the mouth. Typically, the infant will respond by opening her mouth with the tongue protruding on the same side as the area touched.

If this is retained the infant may have drooling and a tongue that sits too forward in the mouth. Children will likely have difficulty with swallowing and chewing in sequence order as well as possible speech and articulation problems because of the dysfunctional tongue. Hypersensitivity around lips and mouth or oral sensitivity can be seen as twitching or not liking foods due to texture.

They may have hypotonic or hypertonic muscle tone, asymmetric muscle patterns or delayed developmental milestones.

Poor manual dexterity may be seen later on as there is a reflex loop between the hand and the mouth seen by kneading movements of the hand associated with suckling.

The Snout Reflex

The Snout Reflex does not start during the pregnancy but after birth and integrates by one year of age. It is related to sucking behaviour. To activate the Snout Reflex lightly tap the baby's/child/adult's upper lip. Muscle contraction around the mouth and base of the nose causes the mouth to pucker or protrude (if not integrated yet), creating the resemblance of an animal snout[clxi].

When retained, it may indicate a myriad of cerebral disorders that affect the frontal lobes and pyramidal tracks. This reflex is often seen retained in children on the autism spectrum. This may also show as a frontal release sign from brain injury from trauma or chemical damage.

The Glabellar Tap

The Glabellar Tap reflex should emerge at birth and integrate at about 4 months of age after birth. It is activated by tapping the forehead between the eyebrows and nose and watching the eyes blink. Repeated tapping should lead to habituation with blinking being suppressed[clxii].

It is suggested that the glabellar tap reflex may have provided an evolutionary/adaptive purpose in infant hominids by protecting the eyes from danger. It appears also to be associated with heightened dopamine/adrenaline response neurologically. Patients with high vigilance commonly demonstrate non-integrated glabellar tap. When integrated, the patient will blink in response to the first several taps and then become habituated to the stimulus by about the fifth tap as the brain processes that the threat the eyes is not imminent. If the subject continues blinking it is called Myerson's sign[clxiii]. Myersons sign is often seen in older patients and is associated with many brain conditions or cerebral pathologies, including, but not limited to Parkinson's disease, cerebral palsy, tumours, and head injury.

As you can see from the above the frontal release signs are really seen when the suppression or integration of the primitive reflexes fails (or never occurs). The six reflexes include the hands-grasping, Babkin palmomental reflex, sucking, rooting, snout reflex, and glabellar tap reflex, all demonstrate poor function of the frontal lobes of the brain if seen in people older than about

12 months of age. All reflexes are associated with infant survival initially but when retained, they will affect sucking and swallowing, speech, and fine motor skills development of the child, which is probably why they have been seen in children on the spectrum, we are highly likely to most of these reflex signs in children and adults with cranio-facia maldevelopment, airway dysfunction and both Posterior and anterior tongue tie.

Sleep and Airway

I hope the reader has now got a greater understanding of the importance of the CNS and that it is a dynamic evolution not a static occurrence, we are not hatched in adult form and that physical dysfunction will affect neurological and emotional development as well as the reverse. Our next section is to appraise you of the importance of airway function and Sleep. Both the phenomena of sleep and the significance of airway patency are imperative to human health, growth, and long-term wellbeing in all aspects. You will die quickly if either are disturbed. The following section will try to explain important aspects of the Continuum, how the beginnings of dysfunction in the infant neonate end up as disease in the adult. The apnoea's and diabetes do not occur courtesy of a deranged fairy with an ill health wand. They are a process that is missed at many stages. The first area to look at is sleep fragmentation, from there we will discuss diseases such as obstructive sleep apnoea, as well as try to give an understanding of how this activates parts of the immune system and causes damage, therefore why airway fragmentation causes sleep fragmentation and how this causes ill health at any age and why this is so important to solve. We will have a brief talk about airway solutions such as CPAP, and mandibular advancement splints and try to round it into an understandable conclusion. One of the concepts I will try to disabuse you of is the idea that conditions just occur, that they are not part of a continuum that starts early on in life and if missed will continue to worse more evolved conditions for example issues will sleep fragmentation, airway and retention of primitive reflexes strongly resemble ADHD, which is diagnosed at 15, or airway fragmentation and tongue tie lead to orthodontic issues, and both can easily become sleep Apnoea.

9

Sleep fragmentation and Apnoea effects in adults:

Our understanding of the nature and consequences of upper-airway obstruction in adults during sleep has evolved considerably over the past two decades. Sleep apnoea is a common sleep disorder that affects millions of people worldwide. It occurs when a person's breathing is interrupted during sleep, leading to poor quality sleep and a range of health problems. While sleep apnoea can affect people of any age, its diagnosis is particularly prevalent in older adults, who are more likely to develop the condition due to a variety of factors, including tongue tie and cranial development issues which is seen by a previous history of orthodontic treatment, as well as weak, floppy, low tone muscle and pharyngeal tissues.

Sleep apnoea, is repeated episodes of obstructive or central apnoea and hypopneas are defined as follows:

Obstructive sleep apnoea is a pause in respiration for more than 10 seconds at least 5 times per hour, due to a blockage of the airway.

There are two types of apnoea, 1. central sleep apnoea (CSA) and 2. obstructive sleep apnoea (OSA). They are differentiated by a lack of respiratory effort in CSA versus continued but ineffective respiratory effort in OSA.

Hypopnea is defined as a reduction in ventilation of at least 50% that results in a decrease in arterial saturation of 4% or more due to partial airway obstruction during sleep[clxiv], together with daytime sleepiness or altered cardiopulmonary function is common[clxv], as we will see changes to circulation due to apnoea and hypopnea is not the end of it.

Apnoea and hypopnea are caused by the airway being sucked closed on inspiration during sleep. During sleep, all muscles relax including the tongue and other muscles in the airway, neck, and throat. This inhibition is associated with alteration in the FPR neurology. In patients with OSA/HS, the dilating muscles can no longer successfully oppose negative pressure within the airway during inspiration which can cause the airway to become narrowed or blocked or collapse.

In people with tongue tie and oral fascial restrictions, the restricted movement of the tongue may contribute to this narrowing or blockage of the airway narrowing the airway space even further. As a result, the person may experience these episodes of interrupted breathing during sleep. The airway is normally kept patent (open) by the dilating muscles. They have higher activity during wakefulness, however during sleep, the muscle tone falls which will naturally allow a degree in airway narrowing.

First Principles • 203

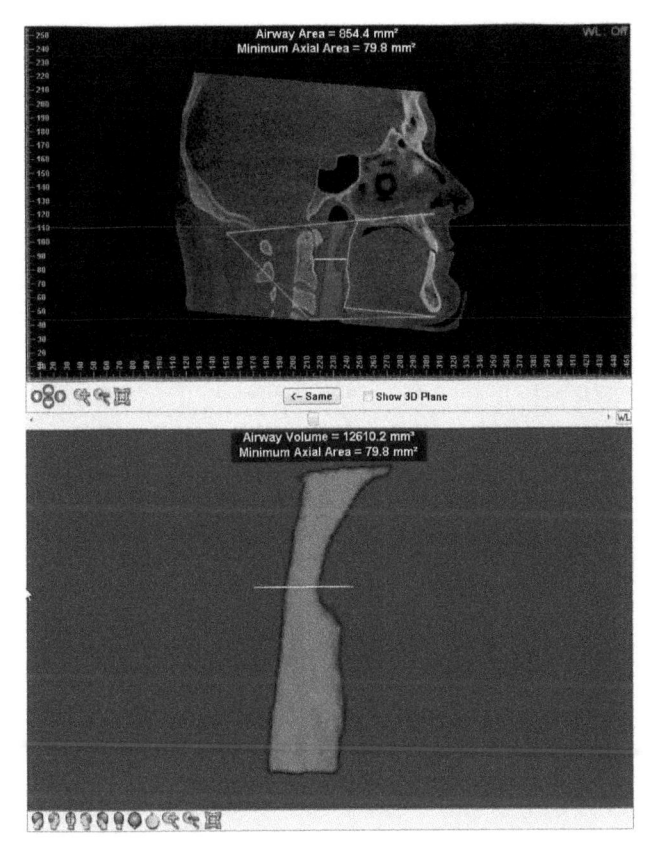

Image 32: 3D CT scan of a lateral head and throat, demonstrating airway width.

THE ABOVE IMAGE shows a narrowed airway with a minimum axial area of only 798 mm^2. This creates greater likelihood of respiratory distress.

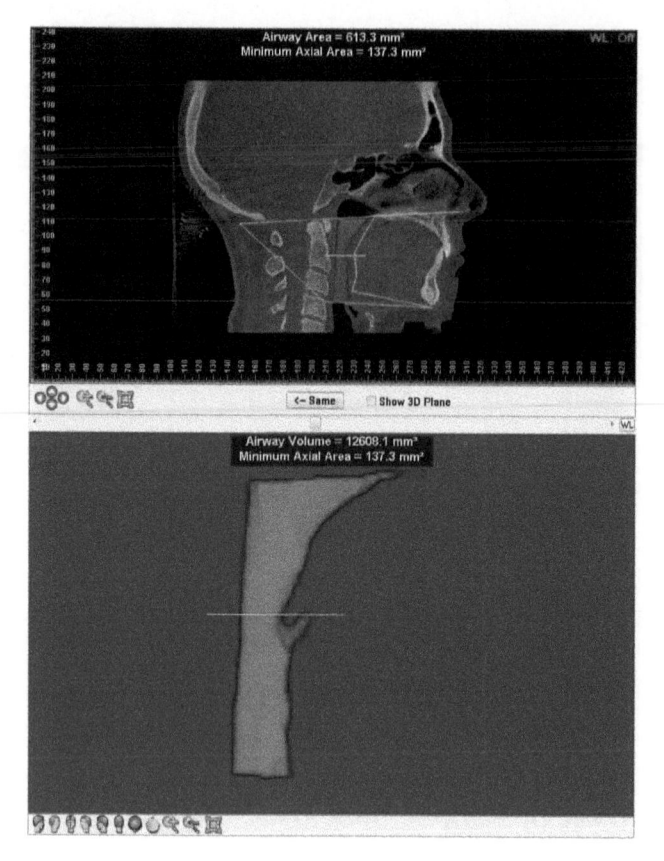

Image 33. Lateral View of a 3D CT scan of the head neck to demonstrate airway width.

The above images shows an airway with a minimal axial area of 137.3 ^{mm2}. The photos allow comparison of two different airways. One has a minimal airway area much smaller than the first, but with very similar airway volumes. The narrowness of the minimal axial area, quite literal creates a significant choke point and narrowing of the airway, making hypopneas and OSA as well as UARS much more likely.

Snoring may then occur followed by airway occlusion and subsequent apnoea; this is most prevalent during REM sleep[clxvi]. The characteristics of this condition include hypoxemia, hypercapnia, intrathoracic pressure swings, surges of systemic blood pressure which are associated with arousals and sleep fragmentation, this has been seen in some severe cases up to 100 times per hour. These characteristics have significant consequences for disease progression which we shall discuss in the next section.

Consequences of OSA - Diseases Associated with Fragmented Sleep

Clearly therefore one of the main risks of sleep apnoea in older adults is an increased risk of cardiovascular disease, simply due to low oxygen, pressure changes and inflammation. Studies have shown that people with sleep apnoea hypoxemia, hypercapnia, will have high blood pressure, as mentioned large intrathoracic pressure swings (up to 120 mm Hg), and surges of systemic blood pressure of up to 250/150 mm Hg which creates significant stress on arterial linings. In some cases, this can create an arterial thickening response and narrowing of the artery, while other negative consequences include aneurysm, stroke, and heart failure[clxvii] and metabolic syndrome.

This is thought to be since sleep apnoea causes intermittent oxygen deprivation, which can damage the cardiovascular system over time. However, give thought to the development of heart disease in younger people which becomes the older adult.

It's probable that airway dysfunction is due to tongue tie or fascial restriction, poor nasal breathing, cranio-facial and jaw maldevelopment (including the impact of orthodontic consequences) and chronic inflammation are actually at the root of or the cause of the whole sleep fragmentation issue which is viewed as subclinical in younger adults and only responded to as the health consequences effect vitality in the older adult.

An interesting paper by Hammond[clxviii] gives weight to our argument, airway fragmentation and sleep fragmentation may be behind the confluence of all of previously mentioned diseases including CHD, stroke, diabetes etc. Hammond found "Death rates from both CHD and stroke were far lower for subjects with neither diabetes nor high blood pressure than for subjects with a history of either of these conditions. In general, subjects with both diabetes and high blood pressure had higher death rates than subjects with just one of these two conditions". We know categorically that OSA, can cause Sleep fragmentation, and sleep fragmentation can cause Diabetes and weight gain which is negatively associated with CHD. We also know that occluded airways in OSA/HS increase blood pressure also strongly associated with CHD, stroke, and negative health consequences. This is another doom loop which is neglected as we treat the hypertension with low-pressure medication and low salt diets, or we treat the diabetes with a drug like metformin and a high fibre diet. What we don't do is consider there may be a physiological cause behind both diseases and that if we don't look for the cause and correct that, the ill health continues. Plenty of people die of heart attacks with low blood pressure, sadly drug therapy for individual risks such as high blood pressure is not well correlated with a reduction in mortality although it may improve arrythmia or the blood pressure[clxix] individually[clxx], the BMJ 2017 paper actually pointed out that the paper did not have enough power to make recommendations, nor were there any prospective studies giving absolute risk only relative risk.

Similarly, we tend to consider diabetes from calories are all equal, so it must be a calorie in versus out imbalance and a lack of will on behalf of the sufferer, rather than a unrecognised physiological issue caused from sleep fragmentation and airway distress. Both can cause an increase in cortisol, which pushes up blood sugar either DiNovo, or from eating and leads to an increase in insulin release, which will have receptor resistance complications and weight gain as a result with a variety of inflammatory metabolic consequences following on.

We don't treat cause only symptoms thus we keep people on the continuum in a doom loop, allowing further complications to occur. This as I'm sure you can imagine is the path to early death or at the very least a cost in enjoyable life years. Our society spends a lot of time desperately clinging to life, holding back the ravages with excessive medical spend. It is estimated that 90% of all health care spending in the medical system is in the last 6 months of peoples lives. With several studies finding " no evidence that higher levels of spending translate into extended survival"[clxxi], let alone better quality of that time. Thus the purpose of this book is to get people to look sooner into the continuum of ill health from airway and sleep fragmentation from all causes, to stop the metabolic and physiological consequences, if at all possible, we need screen programs regularly from year one to grade 10, to catch it before its hard wired in.

OSA Hypopnea and the Mouth Structures

Tongue tie as we have spoken about, is a condition in which the tissue under the tongue at the front or around the root of the tongue at the back, is tight, overly thick, or too short, restricting movement of the tongue and airway stopping the tongue sitting up in the roof of the mouth, creating appropriate anterior thrust. This can cause difficulty swallowing and speaking and has been linked to sleep apnoea.

Other predisposing considerations for OSA and hypopnea include all the factors which cause narrowing of pharynx: this includes obesity (more than 50% of obese patients have body mass index {BMI} greater than 30 kg/m^2), shortening of the mandible or maxilla, shortened cranial bones of the jaw or restrictions to sinus airflow due to septal deviation, or the intrusion of the hard palate into the nasal sinus space as occurs in a narrow high palate termed an adenoid face, issues with sinusitis, rhinitis, and infection in the nasal sinuses fat infiltration of the tongue tissue. Yes, the tongue can have fat deposition in it which of course will thicken it in the mouth and increase the occurrence of occlusion of the airway.

Interestingly, OSA and Hypopneas are a noted cause of obesity and weight gain, due to a myriad of direct and indirect metabolic changes. Which will potentially cause a doom loop if you lay down fat in your tongue. Change in jaw shape may be mild and familial or significant as previously discussed due to teratological issues in the pregnancy, as well as caused by mouth breathing and poor sucking and chewing practices when young.

Hypothyroidism and acromegaly also predispose to OSAHS by narrowing the upper airway with tissue infiltration. Males suffer apnoea more than females, while myotonic dystrophy, Ehlers-Danlos syndrome, and smoking are all risk factors[clxxii].

Other Consequences of OSA and Sleep Fragmentation

Sleep apnoea in older adults presents an increased risk of falls and accidents, especially motor vehicle accidents[clxxiii]. People with sleep apnoea often feel tired and drowsy during the day, which can impair their ability to concentrate and make them more prone to accidents. In fact, apnoea induced somnolence, causes between a 2.45 and sixfold increase in road accidents. Somnolence is particularly dangerous for older adults, who are already at an increased risk of falls due to decreased muscle mass and other age-related changes. CPAP use ≥ 4 h/night was associated with a reduction of MVA incidence (7.6 to 2.5 accidents/1,000 drivers/y). of note in one study it was found that female apnoea suffers were more likely involved in a motor vehicle accident[clxxiv].

Sleep apnoea and sleep fragmentation can also have negative impacts on mental health in everyone let alone older adults. The lack of quality sleep caused by sleep apnoea can lead to feelings of depression and anxiety, as well as memory problems and difficulty with decision making.

Fragmented sleep and sleep-disturbances resulting from sleep disorders such as OSA have been tied to emotional dysregulation and psychiatric disorders[clxxv]. This is one of the potentially nasty consequences for individuals with obstructive sleep apnoea considering that the stress of disturbed sleep results in more or less constant sympathetic arousal. There is strong evidence showing greater risk of depression with abnormal sympathetic arousal responses[clxxvi]. Thus, the overactivation of endocrine responses including the release of adrenaline and corticosteroids to activate wakefulness and protect the airway, has a significant effect on depressive outcomes in patient.

Reported REM sleep abnormalities in depressed patient have mainly included a reduced REM sleep latency and reduced REM-sleep density on polysomnography. They persist after remission of depressive disease; thus, they are considered to represent markers for susceptibility to mood disorders. OSA may affect more than 50% of individuals over the age of 65, and significant depressive symptoms may be present in as many as 26% of a community-dwelling population of older adults. What I'm trying to get at here is that depressive symptoms in the elderly may be as an end result of missed pathology of the head, mouth and airway early in life, causing to sleep fragmentation, leading to a progression of illness.

A recent publication in adolescents, found that increased REM fragmentation was independently associated with higher depression scores. I feel this indicates a high likelihood that the process starts in early life either in utero or infancy due to any of the mentioned reasons, continues through adolescence as it is missed, continues to progress into other disease states and is then picked up finally in later adulthood when symptoms are so gross that they can't be dismissed, either CVD, metabolic syndrome or OSA/HS. Having your sleep disrupted for any reason is really tiring.

Finally, sleep apnoea can also lead to a decreased quality of life in older adults. The constant interrupted sleep and feelings of fatigue can make it difficult for people with the condition to participate in activities they enjoy, leading to a decrease in overall satisfaction with life.

It is important for older adults to be aware of the risks of sleep apnoea and to seek treatment if they suspect they may have the condition. Treatment options for sleep apnoea include devices to provide respiratory support at night such as continuous positive airway pressure (CPAP) therapy, lifestyle changes such as weight loss and quitting smoking, and in some cases, surgery. By addressing sleep apnoea, older adults can improve their overall health and quality of life.

There are several treatment options for sleep apnoea, in addition to continuous positive airway pressure (CPAP) therapy. Some of these options include:

1. Oral appliance therapy: This involves wearing a custom-fit device in the mouth that helps to keep the airway open during sleep.
2. Lifestyle changes: Making changes to your diet and exercise routine, quitting smoking, and avoiding alcohol and sedatives can help to improve symptoms of sleep apnoea.
3. Surgery: In some cases, surgery may be recommended to address underlying causes of sleep apnoea, such as enlarged tonsils or a deviated septum.
4. Positive airway pressure devices: In addition to CPAP, there are other types of positive airway pressure devices that may be recommended, such as bilevel positive airway pressure (BiPAP) or auto-adjusting positive airway pressure (APAP).
5. Oxygen therapy: Supplementing with oxygen during sleep may be helpful for some people with sleep apnoea.
6. Behavioural changes: Making changes to your sleep habits, such as sleeping on your side instead of your back, can help to alleviate symptoms of sleep apnoea.

It's important to note that the most appropriate treatment for sleep apnoea will depend on the individual and the specific cause of their sleep apnoea. It is recommended to speak with a healthcare professional to determine the best course of treatment.

10

Diseases of the Continuum

I would like to give a bit of detail for the lay reader to understand the diseases I am talking about when I mention CVD or diabetes, metabolic syndrome, they are all related to inflammation, sleep fragmentation and airway disturbances. They all can be aggravated and caused by low oxygen states and by tissue acidification. I have tried not to get bogged down by biochemistry and the intricacies of sodium to potassium, blood bicarbonate levels or many other myriad of blood markers to make the book more digestible for the less medically minded, but rest assured sleep fragmentation and airway occlusion alter all of these indirectly and directly. Below we will discuss inflammations effects and constituent parts as it's a word tossed about by many authors and researchers and is not well explained. The thing inflammation is not is a flame like a piece of wood burning, so I will try to make that clearer.

Let's define Cardiovascular Disease (CVD) for a moment. This is a serious collection of conditions that can have many significant negative impacts on a person's health and well-being including an inability to maintain normal life capacity, and in the worst case it can cause early death. The different areas of damage are generally collected under the title heart disease but are made up in 4 main areas':

Types of Cardiovascular Disease

- Coronary Heart Disease
- Stroke
- Peripheral Arterial Disease
- Aortic Disease

Ultimately the impact of all areas of CVD is that it reduces oxygen supply to the tissue at the endpoint of the arterial supply.

Some of the potential negative impacts of heart disease include[clxxvii]:

Heart attacks: heart disease can lead to heart attacks, which can be life-threatening events that require immediate medical attention. A heart attack usually occurs when a blood clot or plaque blocks blood flow to the heart tissue. Without blood, the tissue loses oxygen and dies.

Symptoms include tightness or pain in the chest, neck, back or arms, as well as fatigue, light-headedness, abnormal heartbeat, and anxiety. Women are more likely to have atypical symptoms than men.

Treatment ranges from lifestyle changes and cardiac rehabilitation to medication, stents, and bypass surgery.

Heart failure: heart disease can cause the heart muscle to become weak and unable to pump enough blood to meet the body's needs, leading to heart failure.

Heart failure can occur if the heart cannot pump (systolic) or fill (diastolic) adequately.

Symptoms include shortness of breath, fatigue, swollen legs, and rapid heartbeat.

Treatments can include eating less salt, limiting fluid intake and taking prescription medication. In some cases, a defibrillator or pacemaker may be implanted, to keep the speed and rhythm of the heart muscle regulated.

Angina: Heart disease can cause chest pain or discomfort, known as angina. This is due to reduced blood flow to the heart tissue. Angina is a symptom of coronary artery disease.

Angina feels like squeezing, pressure, heaviness, tightness, or pain in the chest. It can be sudden or recur over time.

Depending on severity, it can be treated by lifestyle changes, medication, angioplasty, or surgery.

Stroke: Heart disease can increase the risk of stroke, which is a serious condition that occurs when the blood supply to the brain is disrupted. Damage to the brain from interruption of its blood supply ensues. This can be minor or more serious, depending on the speed of diagnosis and treatment.

A stroke is a medical emergency.

Symptoms of stroke include trouble walking, speaking, and understanding, as well as paralysis or numbness of the face, arm, or leg.

Early treatment with medication like tPA (clot buster) can minimise brain damage. Other treatments focus on limiting complications and preventing additional strokes.

F.A.S.T.

If you think someone may be having a stroke, act F.A.S.T. and do the following test:

- F—Face: Ask the person to smile. ...
- A—Arms: Ask the person to raise both arms. ...
- S—Speech: Ask the person to repeat a simple phrase. ...
- T—Time: If you see any of these signs, call 9-1-1 right away.

Also Note the time when any symptoms first appear for the assessing physician.

Arrhythmias: Heart disease can cause abnormal heart rhythms, known as arrhythmias, which can be dangerous. Improper beating of the heart, whether irregular, too fast or too slow.

Cardiac arrhythmia occurs when electrical impulses in the heart don't work properly.

There may be no symptoms. Alternatively, symptoms may include a fluttering in the chest, chest pain, fainting or dizziness.

If required, treatment includes anti-arrhythmic drugs, medical procedures, implantable devices, and surgery.

Peripheral Artery Disease: A circulatory condition in which narrowed blood vessels reduce blood flow to the limbs.

Peripheral vascular disease is a sign of fatty deposits and calcium building up in the walls of the arteries called atherosclerosis which is associated with complication of metabolic syndrome. Risk factors include ageing, diabetes, and smoking.

Symptoms may include leg pain, particularly when walking, coldness in the extremities, dry or sweating hands or feet and severe ulcers on the peripheral limbs.

Tobacco cessation, exercise and a healthy diet are often successful treatments. When these changes aren't enough, medication or surgery is used to mitigate signs.

12

Sleep Fragmentation and Diabetes links

Diabetes

From the American centre for disease control (CDC) Diabetes [clxxviii] is a chronic health condition that affects how your body turns food into energy. When your blood sugar goes up, a signal triggers your pancreas to release insulin. Insulin acts like a key to let the blood sugar into your body's cells for use as energy to be used in the Krebs/citric acid cycle. With diabetes, your body doesn't make enough insulin or can't use it as well as it should. When there isn't enough insulin or cells stop responding to insulin termed insulin resistance, too much blood sugar stays in your bloodstream. Over time, that can cause serious health problems, such as obesity, heart disease, vision loss, and kidney disease, cellular glycation and hyperactivation of your immune system creating tissue damage, including neuropathies, eye issues, ulcers and in some cases gangrene.

There is a strong link between OSAHS, sleep fragmentation and diabetes. People with sleep apnoea are significantly more likely to develop diabetes, and people with diabetes are more likely to develop sleep apnoea.

The poor-quality Sleep, sleep fragmentation and OSA is strongly associated with an increased risk of diabetes. This is thought to be since sleep apnoea causes intermittent oxygen deprivation, which can damage the body's ability to regulate blood sugar levels which increases the risk of diabetes. On the other hand, people with diabetes are also more likely to develop sleep apnoea. This is thought to be since high blood sugar levels can damage the nerves and blood vessels that control breathing, leading to sleep apnoea.

Fragmentation of sleep across all stages is associated with a decrease in insulin sensitivity and glucose effectiveness. Increases in sympathetic nervous system and adrenocortical activity likely mediate the adverse metabolic effects of poor sleep quality. Sleep fragmentation led to an increase in morning cortisol levels and a shift in sympathicovagal balance toward an increase in sympathetic nervous system activity and more "stress response". Shifting the sleeper toward increased sympathetic nervous system activity during both sleep and wakefulness. Please keep in mind the release at night in defence of the airway floods the blood stream with adrenocorticoids which don't miraculously stop acting as soon as we wake, they take time to deactivate and detox, they keep acting for hours affect mood motivation and cognitive response in wake time, often these people are diagnosed as generalised anxiety disorder, which makes sense, but is unhelpful as the airway is missed as is the sleep issue except for the difficulty getting to sleep. Drugs are prescribed for that.

Interestingly markers of systemic inflammation and serum adipokines were unchanged with sleep fragmentation, but not so much in OSA, which we will discuss later.

Like OSA, the prevalence of diabetes is also increasing in the United States and worldwide. Type 2 diabetes represents 90-95% of all cases of diabetes. In the past three decades, the number of American adults with diabetes nearly quadrupled with an estimated 29 million people or 9.3% of the population of the United States estimated to have diagnosed or undiagnosed diabetes. Each year, more than 200,000 deaths occur among people with diabetes in the United States making it the country's seventh leading cause of death[clxxix]. Although obesity and ageing are shared risk factors for both OSA and type 2 diabetes, there is growing evidence that the relationship between the two conditions is independent of obesity[clxxx].

Recent data suggest OSA is associated with insulin resistance, independent of obesity.

The association of OSA with diabetes mellitus (DM) is not just due to obesity being common in both conditions. Obesity is associated with DM, and DM may cause vascular and neuropathic damage to the dilator pharyngeal muscles and reduced upper airway sensation; this needs to be further investigated[clxxxi], especially as we have discussed the drive of poor airway function to increase weight gain, and DM risk directly.

Irregular breathing during sleep is also associated with Hepatic dysfunction including the promotion of non-alcoholic fatty liver disease (NAFLD). Non-alcoholic patients with apnoea and hypopnea were found to also have raised liver enzymes and on liver biopsy were found to have fibrosis. This was all independent of body weight[clxxxii]. The good news from the longitudinal data from Wisconsin Sleep Cohort Study indicate that a 10% weight reduction predicts a 26% decrease in the apnoea's or hypopneas[clxxxiii]. So getting slimmer as a therapy should have positive health outcomes.

The question of causality remains as there is a bidirectional association between sleep fragmentation, night-time disordered breathing, and type 2 diabetes. long-standing poorly controlled diabetes can worsen obstructive and central sleep apnoea as well as nocturnal hypoxemia by adversely impacting central control of respiration or upper airway neural reflexes that promote airway patency.

Studies in non-obese young type 1 diabetic sufferers found that they had a high prevalence of OSA and fragmentation. Whereas a study of patient with type 2 diabetes who were hospitalised for intensive glycaemic control therapy found that their night-time glycaemic profile improved significantly (202 ± 65 mg/dL vs. 130 ± 38 mg/dL; $p=0.005$) after 5 days of care[clxxxiv]. This result was accompanied by a 32% reduction in the 4% oxygen desaturation index. This occurred without any change in the subject's body weight or neck circumference, limiting the possibility of easier breathing due to mass reduction, self-reported sleep duration remained unchanged. This says that improvement in blood sugar alone improved oxygenation and improved sleep profiles, regardless of weight, conversely screw up blood sugar and OSA is likely to occur, possibly due to inflammation.

It is important to consider the number of children with increased BMIs, and the significant increase in childhood obesity in western countries, including Australia and New Zealand and the United States of America. We shall use American data since it is a large multicultural cohort and should be suggestive of trends occurring worldwide.

Obesity is defined as a body mass index (BMI) at or above the sex-specific 95th percentile on the US Centres for Disease Control and Prevention (CDC) BMI-for-age growth charts.

Extreme obesity is defined as a BMI at or above 120% of the sex-specific 95th percentile on the CDC BMI-for-age growth charts. Detailed estimates are presented for 2011-2014. The analyses of linear trends in prevalence were conducted using 9 survey periods. Trend analyses between 2005-2006 and 2013-2014 also were conducted. In this nationally representative study of US children and adolescents aged 2 to 19 years, the prevalence of obesity in 2011-2014 was 17.0% and extreme obesity was 5.8%. Between 1988-1994 and 2013-2014, the prevalence of obesity increased until 2003-2004 and then decreased in children aged 2 to 5 years, increased until 2007-2008 and then levelled off in children aged 6 to 11 years, and increased among adolescents aged 12 to 19 years[clxxxv].

From a 2018 paper by Skinner et al, I found "Despite previous reports that obesity in children and adolescents has remained stable or decreased in recent years, we found no evidence of a decline in obesity prevalence at any age. In contrast, we report a significant increase in severe obesity among children aged 2 to 5 years since the 2013–2014 cycle, a trend that continued upward for many subgroups"[clxxxvi].

Previously reported improvements seen in younger children were either an anomaly or transient because national data presented here demonstrate a sharp increase from the last cycle.

The obvious concern that we should be thinking about is the link between this increase in childhood obesity, Sleep fragmentation/OSA and the increase in tongue tie, and cranial maldevelopment as noted by the significant increase in orthodontic therapy in a similar age group. Which is the chicken which is the egg. We constantly hear the ills of child health blamed on bad diet and sedentary lifestyle, but no investigation of airway or sleep fragmentation seems forthcoming. I have seen very hyper obese 4-year-old in my practice, who eat a reasonable diet, don't sit still, or have much screen time, yet are still overweight. The consequences of the weight can be lifelong, losing the weight alone does not seem to stop long term risk of disease. We need a better screening program for kids.

In summary it is important for people with sleep apnoea and/or diabetes to be aware of the link between the two conditions and to seek treatment for both conditions to improve overall health and quality of life. Lifestyle changes have been shown to help, this may include diet change, weight loss, stopping alcohol consumption, reducing sugar intake, while treatment for diabetes may include medication, as well as lifestyle changes, and blood sugar monitoring. In my opinion the focus needs to be on maintaining airway patency and improving quality of the sleep to stop the insulin resistance drive and inflammation in the background that derails the metabolism. This has to be more than a mandibular advancement splint or a CPAP machine.

Inflammation and OSA

Sleep apnoea has been linked to inflammation in the body. Inflammation is a normal immune response to injury or infection, but chronic inflammation can lead to a range of health problems.

As we have been discussing sleep apnoea is a condition that occurs when a person's breathing is interrupted during sleep, leading to poor quality sleep and a range of health problems. One potential health problem associated with sleep apnoea is chronic inflammation. This is thought to be due to the intermittent oxygen deprivation and increased stress on the body caused by sleep apnoeas and or hypopneas (which we will collectively refer to as SA).

Studies have shown that people with SA have higher levels of inflammatory markers in their blood, indicating a state of chronic inflammation. This chronic inflammation has been linked to an increased risk of a range of health problems, including cardiovascular disease, diabetes, and mental health issues.

Definition and discussion of what inflammation is

Inflammation is a process that occurs in response to tissue damage or infection. It is characterized by a range of signs and symptoms, including swelling, redness, heat, pain, and loss of function. Inflammation is a normal and necessary part of the body's immune response, as it helps to protect against harmful stimuli and promotes healing. However, chronic, or persistent inflammation can contribute to the development of various diseases, such as cancer, heart disease, and autoimmune disorders.

The hallmark signs of inflammation are known as the "four cardinal signs," which are swelling, redness, heat, and pain. These signs are caused by the accumulation of fluid, immune cells, and other substances in the affected area. The swelling is caused by the accumulation of fluid, which can press on nerve endings and cause pain. The redness is caused by increased blood flow to the affected area, which brings immune cells and other substances to the site of injury or infection. The heat is caused by increased blood flow and the metabolic activity of immune cells.

There are several different types of inflammation, including acute and chronic inflammation. Acute inflammation is a short-term response that occurs within hours or days of tissue damage or infection. It is characterized by a rapid and intense response that helps to protect against further harm and promotes healing. Chronic inflammation, on the other hand, is a long-term response that can last for weeks, months, or even years. It is often associated with ongoing or recurrent tissue damage or infection, and it can contribute to the development of various diseases.

Inflammation is a complex process that involves the activation of various immune cells and signalling pathways. One way that immune cells are classified is based on their production of cytokines, which are small proteins that help to coordinate immune responses. The main cytokines involved in inflammation are produced by T helper cells, which are a type of immune cell that help to activate and coordinate other immune cells.

There are three main types of T helper cells that are involved in immune responses: TH1 cells, TH2 cells, and TH3 cells. Each of these types of T helper cells produces a different set of cytokines that help to regulate immune responses in different ways.

TH1 cells produce cytokines such as interferon-gamma and IL-2, which help to activate immune cells such as macrophages and natural killer cells. These immune cells are important for fighting viral infections and for activating the immune response to intracellular pathogens.

TH2 cells produce cytokines such as IL-4, IL-5, and IL-13, which help to activate immune cells such as eosinophils and basophils. These immune cells are important for fighting helminth (worm) infections and for activating the immune response to allergens.

TH3 cells are responsible for suppressing immunological responses and promoting tolerance to self-antigens through the production of cytokines including transforming growth factor-beta (TGF-beta). The TH3 cell is hypothesised to have a role in immune response modulation and in the avoidance of autoimmune reactions and excessive inflammation.

The transforming growth factor beta is essential for preventing unwanted immunological reactions. Other immune cells, such as T-helper cells, B cells, and natural killer cells, have their activation and proliferation stymied by TGF-beta.

Tolerance, or the immune system's capacity to tell self from non-self, is maintained in part by TH3 cells, which are also involved in this process. Many autoimmune and inflammatory illnesses, such as multiple sclerosis, inflammatory bowel disease, and rheumatoid arthritis, have been associated to TH3 cell dysregulation.

Further study is needed to completely understand the roles and possible therapeutic uses of TH3 cells, although it is crucial to remember that the role of TH3 cells in the immune system is still being investigated.

As part of the inflammatory response, various cytokines and other cell signalling molecules are produced and released, which help to coordinate and amplify the immune response.

IL-6 is a cytokine that is produced by a variety of cell types, including immune cells, endothelial cells, and fibroblasts. It is a pleiotropic cytokine, which means that it has multiple functions. During inflammation, IL-6 is produced in response to various stimuli, such as tissue damage or infection. It helps to activate immune cells such as T cells and B cells, and it also plays a role in the development of fever and the acute phase response. I consider it the fast responder, who turns up to the party (wound, infection or damage site) first and signals to all the other immune response cells to come join in. It is capable of epigenetic modification and in some people can be overexpressed, leaving them likely to have a greater or elongated inflammatory response.

TNF-alpha (TNF-a) is a cytokine that is produced by a variety of immune cells, including macrophages, T cells, and natural killer cells. It is a key mediator of inflammation, and it plays a role in activating immune cells, inducing fever, and promoting the acute phase response. TNF-a is also involved in the regulation of various immune and inflammatory responses, such as apoptosis (programmed cell death), angiogenesis (the formation of new blood vessels), and tissue repair. TNF-a is a likely cause of peripheral vascular or nerve damage in conditions such as diabetes, as the body uses glycation (from excess sugar) to signal when it's time for the immune system to kill the cell as its starting to get old, this is what is meant by apoptosis. This is actually the basis for the hbA1c test which measures the amount of glucose attached to red cell haemoglobin. We consider it to determine if you're a well-controlled or bad diabetic. However, think big picture, we developed across many hundreds of millennia in a low sugar/carbohydrate environment, we can now consume a year's worth of sugar in a matter of days. The consequence of which is excessive glycation and activation of apoptosis, faster than the body can repair the tissue, this creases the doom loops leading to neuropathy and peripheral vascular damage in diabetes and metabolic syndrome, let alone the kidneys.

C-reactive protein (CRP) is a protein that is produced by the liver in response to inflammation. It is part of the acute phase response, which is a group of physiological changes that occur in response to inflammation or tissue damage. CRP levels in the blood can be measured as a marker of inflammation, and high levels of CRP are often found in people with infections or other inflammatory conditions. It is used as a stand-in for IL6 which is less easy to measure and will be driven higher by NAFLD.

NF-kappaB (NF-kB) is a transcription factor that is involved in the regulation of gene expression. It is activated in response to various stimuli, such as inflammation, stress, and oxidative stress. Activation of NF-kB leads to the production of various cytokines and other signalling molecules that are involved in the immune response.

In summary TH1 cells, TH2 cells, and TH3 cells are different types of T helper cells that produce different sets of cytokines and help to regulate immune responses in different ways. TH1 cells are important for activating immune responses to viral infections and intracellular pathogens, TH2 cells are important for activating immune responses to helminth(parasite) infections and allergens, and TH3 cells help to suppress immune responses and promote tolerance to self-antigens.

IL-6, TNF-a, CRP, and NF-kB are all molecules that are involved in the immune response to inflammation. IL-6 is a cytokine that helps to activate immune cells and is involved in the development of fever and the acute phase response. TNF-a is a cytokine that is involved in activating immune cells and regulating various immune and inflammatory responses. CRP is a protein that is produced by the liver in response to inflammation and is a marker of the acute phase response. NF-kB is a transcription factor that is activated in response to various stimuli and regulates the production of cytokines and other signalling molecules involved in the immune response.

Sleep Apnoea causes chronic ill health.

I want to raise the potential mechanism by which sleep apnoea may cause chronic health consequences. I have alluded to it through the book, this being through immune hyperactivation. Some studies have shown that people with sleep apnoea have increased levels of immune markers, such as C-reactive protein (CRP) and proinflammatory cytokines[clxxxvii], (like those we discussed above), compared to people without sleep apnoea. These markers are associated with inflammation, chronic inflammation and have been linked to a number of diseases, including heart disease[clxxxviii], stroke[clxxxix], and diabetes[cxc].

As we have discussed, there are several potential mechanisms by which sleep apnoea may lead to immune activation and inflammation. For example, sleep apnoea (and hypopneas) can cause repetitive episodes of hypoxia (low oxygen levels) and oxidative stress, which can damage cells and stimulate the immune response. Sleep apnoea may also disrupt the normal sleep-wake cycle, which can affect the body's ability to regulate immune responses. Additionally, sleep apnoea may lead to changes in gut microbiota, which can affect the immune system.

The immune system's response to inflammation involves the release of a variety of immune cells and signalling molecules, including interleukin 6 (IL-6), tumour necrosis factor alpha (TNF-alpha), and C-reactive protein (CRP). These molecules help to coordinate the immune response and promote healing, but if they are produced in excess or for prolonged periods of time, they can contribute to chronic inflammation. In addition to these molecules, the activation of the nuclear factor kappa-light-chain-enhancer of activated B cells (NF-kappaB) pathway is specifically linked to inflammation. NF-kappaB as we spoke about above has been implicated in the development of various inflammatory diseases.

Now for something completely different, there is another vector driving OSA, hypertension and sleep disruption, and it's not us. The gut houses the biome which is a collection of bacteria, fungi, parasites and viruses that drive around in us like a car. They are not us and while they may share the space with us they are not us and may not share the same goals as we have. They can create pathology and tissue damage, including the release of endotoxins and influence the levels of immune activation of the gut. Activated lymphoid tissue (GALT). Technically the bacteria are not in us but exist on the endothelial lining or skin on the lining of the digestive tract, the luminal space, which arguably is no more inside us than the hole is inside a donut.

The gut biome is involved with OSA and CVD, and other pathologies, there is evidence of bidirectionality that chemicals released by the biome drive the brain to bring about OSA, notwithstanding that the inflammatory stress and endocrine dysfunction impacts the gut health, the brush border integrity and can cause the death of commensal bacteria, leaving less savoury types behind that can live in a less hospitable environment. This comes back to Dr Louis Pastuer's final statement on his deathbed, " la Milieu" not the bacteria that makes the difference. Medical science has tried hard not to listen to this concept and have focused on the bacteria as the cause of all ills. Where I think it's likely a combination of both these thoughts that lead to issues. It's clear that in one host a bacteria can cause great harm, and the same species in another causes no issues, thus there must be something to the milieu and some signalling device such as interaction with the immune system in the host that makes the difference.

Gut microbiota OSA and hypertension

In a direction that many would not consider a surprise, the gut bacteria exert a significant effect on hypertension and OSA. Experiments in germ free mice show that they have low blood pressure, when compared to regular mice. This raises the suspicion that factors to do with the interaction of the gut microbiota with the host gut wall, and gut immune system have an impact on the creation of hypertension[cxci]. Gut bacteria including *Anaerobic bacteria, Bifidobacterium, Lactobacillus,* and *Streptococcus*, produce SCFAs, (short chain fatty acids), which interface with the gut wall processes and appear to regulate adipogenesis (weight gain), reactivity of the immune system, as well as sensitivity to insulin, indicating that the output of bacteria have a significant interplay with the potential for disease pathogenesis.

SCFA receptors are found distributed across many cell tissue types, including those in the intestinal epithelium, adipose cells, pancreatic islet cells, T cells (immune response cells as we discussed), along with sympathetic nerve cells. From this we can deduce that the bacteria that produce the SCFAs are capable of modifying the health and function of the nervous system and the immune system, and could have a hand in issues of obesity and diabetes amongst others. SCFAs produced by intestinal bacteria have been shown to help in maintaining blood pressure stability and immune system homeostasis at normal physiological concentrations, moreover, propionate also protects from hypertensive end-organ damage[cxcii].

The point being is that dysbiosis (meaning a loss of beneficial microbial (another term for bacterial) input or signal and an expansion of pathogenic or opportunistic microbes), can alter how the immune system operates the connected end organs such as the cardiovascular system and blood supply and have been shown to increase hypertension in them. Dysbiosis is thought to trigger pro-inflammatory effects and immune dysregulation associated with various disease states, including non-alcoholic steatohepatitis[cxciii] (fatty liver disease) which is a key indicator of diabetes /metabolic syndrome and is associated with OSA, obesity, and is seen in patients with sleep fragmentation.

Changes in the microbiome have been observed in many diseases, including inflammatory bowel disease (IBD), type 2 diabetes, obesity, psychiatric disorders, asthma, and cardiovascular disease. Gut dysbiosis with all their metabolites have been observed in patients with hypertension and OSA. Consider the bidirectionality of this, which causes what? OSA causes bacterial dysbiosis leading to downstream effects or the dysbiosis leads to changes that cause OSA?

Some of the hallmarks of OSA include sleep fragmentation and chronic intermittent hypoxia. This increases activation of the sympathetic and renin-angiotensin-sin-aldosterone system (RASS) and insufficiency of blood supply to systemic organs including the kidneys, heart, genitals as well as obvious ones including the feet, as blood is diverted to survival tissues, such as the heart pump, lungs and skeletal muscles for fighting or running, even when asleep. These are all areas associated with capillary bed damage in diabetes and CVD.

Intermittent hypoxia also leads to damage to the mucosal lining of the gut by way of ischemia then reperfusion. This creates an acidic anaerobic environment which favours non commensal bacteria that thrive in lower oxygen milieu. This can alter the ratio of Firmicutes to Bacteroides in the biome. The F:B is considered by many researchers as an indicator of gut health and vibrancy and affects the integrity of the gut mucosal barrio, that keeps the outside world from getting into the body proper.

The Bacteroides phylum has been associated with production of SCFA that are anti-inflammatory and increase mucosal barrier integrity, thus a loss of Bacteroides and an increase in the F:B ratio can lead to situations termed leaky gut[cxciv] which has associated malabsorption, nutritional dysfunction, upregulation of mast cells in defence of the body. Not only this, but there appears to be a gut microbiota disruption leading to cross talk between the brain function via the microbiota–gut–brain axis that is specific to OSA/HS sufferers which is led by Ruminococcus, and Prevotella. Thus, there is a possibility that poor eating and lifestyle habits upregulates alterations in the bacterial subtypes in the gut, leading to sleep fragmentation enhancing the outcome towards OSA/HS.[cxcv]

We know that damage to the epithelial lining and damage to the tight and gap junctions activates an immune response and alters nutritional absorption to the body. Indications of this are seen as irritable bowel disease and, in some instances, can progress to more serious disorders such as atherosclerosis[cxcvi] and inflammatory bowel disease[cxcvii]. As by now I hope we are all aware these diseases are driven by inflammatory activation and progression, and in the case of plaques, the intermittent hypoxia accelerated growth and vulnerability of atherosclerotic plaque, which probably acted by triggering the activation of proinflammatory TLR4/NF-κB signalling[cxcviii], these risks and outcomes were particularly obvious in chronic severe OSA patients.

As noted, hypoxia syndromes including OSA have significant consequences for the mucosal epithelium due to ischemia. There is a relationship between the chronicity of the ischemia and the amount of damage occurring. This is demonstrated by Plasma intestinal fatty acid binding protein (I-FABP)[cxcix]. I-FABP is a small protein released into circulation when intestinal wall membrane integrity is lost and is a highly sensitive marker of ischemic damage to intestinal mucosa. Studies have demonstrated the reliability of the levels of I-FABP found in OSA patients correlating with the ischemic reperfusion injury to the intestinal mucosa. That levels are significantly higher than controls in OSA/HS patients, and that this blood marker may be a useful indicator to monitor success of treatment or severity of disease in OSA/HS patients.

To summarise, we can see that there is a link between the gut microbiota and negative consequences in OSA/HS patients. Studies have suggested a bidirectional crosstalk where problems in the biome drive sleep fragmentation which leads to obesity and diabetes which are noted risk factors for OSA/HS. However, Patients with OSA/HS are noted to have inflammatory upregulation which is associated with driving gut microbiota dysregulation.

So, let's take it back a step to our earlier discussion on how we got here. Previously we discussed that open mouth breathing in infants led to atopy, inflammation, asthma, and dermatitis as per this quote "In conclusion, this study demonstrated that mouth breathing is a risk factor for AD development, especially in children with a genetic family history of AD and can be a risk factor for tonsillitis (tonsillar hypertrophy) and class II dental malocclusion. Furthermore, mouth breathing during sleep (MBS) was closely related to allergic diseases and other respiratory diseases. Therefore, MBS is expected to be more harmful to children than MBD[cc]. We can further draw your attention to this situation being correlated with or causative of reflux in infants [cci]. Katz et als work shows strong links with snoring and OSA in infants with reflux. In the literature this reflux is called colic and that Colic is linked with gut inflammation (as determined by faecal calprotectin) and dysbiosis, independent of mode of feeding, with fewer *Bifidobacilli*[ccii].

Thus, we can see that there is a pathway to get from mouth breathing to gut dysbiosis that starts in the newborn. This makes me more certain that the early life breathing maladaptation's, which are associated with primitive reflex retention and heightened stress/startle responses leads on to gut dysbiosis and sets the child up for a lifetime of ill health and disease that is diagnosed generally after 40 years of age as diabetes, obesity heart disease and many other physical ills, as well as neurocognitive impairment, including ADHD, anxiety, OCD, and depression to name a few variants.

MCAS

Mast cell activation syndrome and Sleep/airway fragmentation

Mast cell activation syndrome is an autoimmune condition of massive significance. The most major reason is that it is largely hidden and considered to be many other conditions. This is because Mast cell activation syndrome (MCAS) appears to be a extraordinarily heterogeneous chronic multisystem polymorbidity of general themes of chronic Inflammation (the "universal constant of the disease) allergic-type phenomena (e.g. allergy, urticaria, angioedema, anaphylaxis) aberrant growth/development in potentially any tissue (e.g., cysts, fibrosis, aneurysms, weak and abnormal connective tissue (such as Ehlers-Danlos syndrome and possibly tongue tie), ? neurodevelopmental disorders (autism)) ...the far dominant "bulk" of the iceberg of mast cell activation disease (MCAD)[i].

Owing to the tremendous variability of the complete spectrum of clinical manifestations in such people, the diagnosis of this disease is confounding for the practitioner, much alone the patient living with it. The physiology of MCAS means that the condition itself, which is caused by the same overactivated Mast cells in each person, releases a variety of chemical mediators, in fact over 1000 are noted, not just the two most commonly associated with mastocytosis, including histamine and tryptase. Symptoms can wax and wane, and migrate through the body, partially because of the mast cell's ability to cross talk with the bloodstream as well as the nervous system. Typically, signs will include flushing, allergic-type issues, fatigue, dermato-graphism, cognitive dysfunction, irritated eyes/nose/mouth/ throat,

As you can see, there are several symptoms that can develop in various systems and locations of the body. MCAS is a tragedy because it falls into the continuum pattern. Meaning that it is commonly diagnosed as a single condition by the examiner, via the prism of their specialisation. What I mean is that an immunologist will see the IgE allergy and treat for that, or they may present with blood clots at a haematologist. Without either specialist realising it was caused by the same cells. As a result, the true illness is misdiagnosed or underdiagnosed.

From an evolutionary point of view mast cells are thought to have developed over 500 million years ago and may have served as the original prototype neuroimmune-endocrine cell to protect us. They evolved into a master regulator of such interactions, especially as most of the known diseases involve neuroinflammation that worsens with stress[ii], which we will discuss soon.

Mast cells are technically hematopoietic tissue immune cells. They are found in neuroendocrine organs in the brain such as the hypothalamus, pineal, pituitary, as well as the ovaries, uterus, and pancreas where their function is currently unknown, but we can see their negative aspects by way of conditions such as dysmenorrhea, autism, Parkinson's disease, dementia, and many others. Mast cells have historically related to allergies because of their high histamine and tryptase content, but more recently with immunity and inflammatory control due to the production and release of several cytokines and chemokines. Mast cells are found perivascularly and express numerous receptors for various ligands such as allergens, pathogens, neurotransmitters, neuropeptides, and hormones such as acetylcholine, calcitonin gene-related peptide (CGRP), corticosteroids, corticotropin-releasing hormone (CRH), -endorphin, epinephrine, 17-oestradiol, gonadotrophins (VIP), in fact over 200 different receptors have been found on mast cells.

Moreover, MC can produce and release the majority of its neurohormonal triggers, including ACTH, CRH, endorphins, HKA, leptin, melatonin, NT, SP, and VIP, leading to mimicry of many diseases, including pseudo allergies.

Animal studies have demonstrated that the number of diencephalic MC increases during courtship in doves, but stimulation of brain and nasal MC activates the hypothalamic-pituitary-adrenal (HPA) axis. Current data suggests that MC reactivity varies during the day, and it's worth noting that melatonin appears to control MC output. Nevertheless, the mechanism by which MC modify their phenotype or preferentially release certain chemicals in different pathological situations is still unclear.

Mast cells arose around 500 million years ago and may have functioned as the initial prototype neuro-immuno-endocrine cell before evolving into a master regulator of such interactions, particularly given that most known disorders involve neuroinflammation that increases with stress.

In clinical practice neurologists and psychiatrists frequently encounter patients whose central and/or peripheral neurologic and/or psychiatric symptoms (NPS) are accompanied, persistently or episodically, by a variety of other multi-system symptoms for which investigation often finds no cause and for which empiric therapy often provides little to no benefit When one considers the triggering of pathologically hyperexcitable mast cell (MC) by neuropeptides corticotropin-releasing hormone (CRH) and neurotensin[iii], it becomes likely that the intensity of mast cell activation disease (MCAD) symptoms is regularly modulated by psychologically stressful situations and that Doctors not experienced with MCAS/D can misinterpret MCAD symptoms as somatization, being "its all in your head".

How does MCAS relate to Airway and sleep fragmentation?

Dr Larry Afrin a noted researcher in the MCAS field, has noted many MCAS patients have sleep apnoea as a diagnosed comorbidity prior to MCAS diagnosis.

"The apnoea type is almost always obstructive, is found in 15% of MCAS patients and curiously occurs not uncommonly in non-obese patients, raising questions of mechanisms which might include airways narrowed by oedema, hypertrophy, fibrosis, or excessive mucus, or excessive loss of airway muscular tone in sleep"[iv].

Afrin's finding draws a direct connection to the concepts proposed in the continuum. Failures in REM sleep, due to the retained FPR, lead to over paralysis of the airway muscles and is noted to cause non obstructive sleep apnoea.

The work in the MCAS field shows that chemical mediators in mast cells are bidirectional, between the nervous system and the immune system, and especially via the bloodstream.

There are several important things to consider here: we know that sleep fragmentation drives inflammation, secondly, we know that airway fragmentation and mouth breathing leads to sleep fragmentation.

Further we know that there are epigenetic alterations in children who have midline oral fascial restrictions, which may include a greater propensity to Mast cell activation.

Discussion with Doctor Afrin elucidated a couple of interesting points,

1. That it's not the amount of mast cells that makes the difference, but the degree of hyperactivation that makes the difference. The more activated, the easier it is to drive degranulation and release one of a 1000 different possible chemical combinations. T
2. The second major point I learned is that mast cells derive from pleuropoetic bone marrow cells in different parts of the body, can be activated in different ways in different areas of the body,
3. Patients with MCAS can assimilate epigenetic faults into stem cell lines leading to MCAS. This brings us back to 1 carbon folate B12 SAMe metabolism which is also intrinsically linked to issues with tongue tie. Dr Afrin's point was that the patient may have started with normal cell lines and inculcated a fault into a stem cell of a mast cell during cellular replication, due to some threat or stressor leading to the change in activation sensitivity.

Given the mast cells phenomenal capacity for binding receptors and releasing so many mediators, they have an almost infinite capacity to create issues in the human body, mimic almost any disease and present in non-conforming ways. Commonly overlooked is what their purpose is and how they cross talk with different cell tissue types.

From Professor Pete Smith's work we know that mast cells are sentinel cells that are there to protect us. We find them at what he calls guardian sites, places where threat occurs:

- Hands
- Feet
- Face
- Oral mucosal surfaces

They are in places where the outside and inside worlds meet, think bowel vagina, urethra, nose, and lungs. Further they are in discs and connective tissues especially around joints. They do not work alone and interplay with sensory nerves, eosinophils, enteroendocrine cells, CD4 lymphocyte cells as well as epithelial cells.

Think about this work from the point of view of threat to survival. The activated Mast cells can be part of a doom loop that is capable of potentiating OSA[v]. Hypoxia results in OSA and is noted to induce mast cells to release IL6, while not appearing to release other cytokines. The Mast cells are stable in this situation and don't degranulate in hypoxic conditions, in response to changes in pH, they are considered to have an important function in innate responses to inflammation and bacteria, virus, and parasite infections, this would make sense considering how early in our evolution they arose. If you consider low oxygen environments in a lung filled with mucus, infection will have the upper hand, but our mast cells are there to save the day and clear the pathogen.

Mast cells are phenomenally robust, and can even survive gamma radiation; in fact, some papers show that radiation and electromagnetic frequencies can actually potentiate mast cells. There are also several studies on the role of mast cells in ischemia and reperfusion injury, e.g., myocardial infarction, and in hyponea. Mast cell degranulation has been shown in models of ischemia- reperfusion models, (which snoring and hypopnea mimics as against true apnoea), but from indirect route not just the hypoxia[vi]. Interestingly people with normal mast cell lines done have significant degranulation of mast cells in response to hypoxia, in fact they respond to HIF-1a independent manner to downregulating the release of proinflammatory cytokines like TNF-α, thereby avoiding uncontrolled degranulation, which could lead to excessive inflammation and severe tissue damage, which is exactly the opposite of what occurs in MCAS patients as well as in patients with chronic midline brain stem issues involved with retained primitive reflexes and oral fascial restriction as we have discussed.

Further we know that mast cells are essential for the development of hypoxia induced retinopathy. The activation of mast cells by relative hypoxia but not hyperoxia is via the TRPA1 ion channel. As such TRPA1 can therefore be considered an oxygen sensor that induces mast cell degranulation. TRPA1 is a primarily ion channel sensor of noxious stimuli and is sensitive to changes in oxygen tension. Although it has previously been shown that relative hypoxia after exposure to hyperoxia altered the expression of a diverse set of hypoxia-regulated genes, we clearly demonstrate that mast cells can trigger an "angiogenic switch" in retinopathy[vii].

It is interesting that it is not the initial change from low to high oxygen concentrations, but rather the subsequent relative hypoxia that triggers mast cell degranulation. Think of this in the sense of chronic snoring, and the volume of adult-onset eye disease. From a treatment practicality point of view, we know that TRPA1 reactivity. Issues can be calmed by menthol and CBD in the right doses.

Otolaryngologist Lewis Newberg MD, provided more information about threat response leading to OSA and the neuro-immuno-endocrine aspects of mast cells. His work found that OSA is driven by exposure to environmental pollutant particulates from the environment leading to increased mast cell activation in the ethmoid mucosal tissue[viii]. His work found that leptin is independently associated with OSA, regardless of obesity status, but that patients with OSA have greater fat deposition that non apnoeic patients, which is deposited in places like the central throat versus the abdominal.

Current findings indicate that the neuropeptide leptin has a much larger physiological function than only regulating body weight and energy consumption. Leptin, for example, has been shown to impact fertility, angiogenesis, and immunological function. Leptin increases platelet aggregation in vitro and is required for the creation of persistent thrombi in vivo. These actions are mediated by platelet leptin receptors. Chronic hyperleptinemia, on the other hand, is now thought to have a role in the aetiology of several types of obesity-related hypertension[ix], all of which occurs in OSA as discussed earlier. These latter findings, along with the findings of the current investigation, suggest the idea that leptin may promote, or at least play a role in the development of, hypertension and cardiovascular disease in OSA patients, possibly promoted by MCAS.

To bring this further into the sphere of the continuum, In the presence of obesity, leptin insufficiency is related with higher PaCO2 and hypoventilation. It has been proven that infusion of leptin enhances the ventilatory responses of leptin-deficient ob/ob mice. The stimulating impact of leptin on ventilation is irrespective of weight, carbon dioxide generation, and food consumption, indicating that leptin has a direct influence on the brain's respiratory control centres. A study in mice found that "Three days of leptin infusion (30 μ g/d) markedly increased minute ventilation across all sleep/wake states, but particularly during rapid eye movement (REM) sleep when respiration was otherwise profoundly depressed. The effect of leptin was independent of food intake, weight, and CO_2 production, indicating a reversal of hypoventilation by stimulation of central respiratory control centres"[x]. As we can see the mast cell mediators have an interesting role in regulating REM breathing phase, which also links in with issues of the FPR and threat response.

Dr Newberg's comments on restless leg syndrome (RLS) in OSA patients gives us another important clue in how MCAS is involved in threat induced breathing dysfunction. "RLS has specific brain receptors for neural misfiring to legs. The reduction in leptin or the increase of the mean oxygen level in successful OSA surgery reduces RLS symptoms. Neuropeptide Y (NPY) and leptin are increased in spinal fluid affecting inputs and outputs to neurons by controlling synapses in the hypothalamus and regulating respiration".

Upper airway resistance syndrome is a stage of OSA that is characterised by severe daytime drowsiness and normal RDI. Patients with UARS experience snoring and persistent mouth breathing due to nasal blockage and airway resistance, which is accompanied by an increase in EEG arousals. There is a strong chance that hypothalamic neuropeptides usually associated with release from the hypothalamus influence particular receptor sites and modify neuronal circuit activity.

But…. what if all these chemicals were able to be released from mast cells in the first place. This would mean that the increased threat response, real or imagined, would drive an increase in sentinel mast cells, which become more sensitive to activation, and release more mediators that can drive brain dysregulation including leptin, neuropeptide Y and many others. According to work by Wei-Can Chen[xi], mast cells absolutely can release NPY which makes a degree of sense. NPY acts as an immunomodulatory chemical and can act to inhibit NK cell activation, thus trying to stop excess inflammation, among other functions.

The point being is that dysfunction in the pregnancy can set the child up for midline structural faults that drive mouth breathing which is strongly associated with an increase in inflammation and atopy, bringing us to the beginning of the continuum.

The retention of FPR leads to REM fragmentation and an increase in what later becomes recognised as anxiety which drives potentiation of mast cell production, that accumulate in the guardian sites and start cross talk as part of the drive to increase organism survival.

The repetition of threat upon threat increases the activation of the system leading to accumulation of symptoms, and a worsening of health.

Animal models suggest that the cytokine interleukin-1 (IL-1), which has pleiotropic effects such as sleep induction, fever, anorexia, hypotension, immunomodulation, and pituitary hormone release, is a plausible mediator for MP's sleep-inducing actions. In rabbits, cats, rats, and monkeys, IL-1 delivered intravenously, intracerebroventricularly, or locally to brain stem regions resulted in an increase in SWS and suppression of REM sleep. Rats demonstrated greater circadian sensitivity to the effects of IL-1. We know categorically that Mast cells can release IL1 along with IL33, both of which create inflammation in psoriasis[xii].

Normal but aged participants were observed to exhibit increased host defence activation during sleep, accompanied by the expected decrease in REM sleep, but no changes in NREM sleep or SWS. Like with individuals with advanced infections, the apparent inability of somnogenic cytokines to improve sleep in the elderly may be due to central nervous system degradation, lower sensitivity to cytokines, or both. Conversely, the apparent correlations between sleep and cytokines may not be due to intrinsic linkages between sleep-wake behaviour and host defence mechanisms, but rather to the impacts of circadian rhythm, thermoregulation, and/or neuroendocrine system disturbances. Induced by mast cells, likely a response to the sleep fragmentation. Work by Moldofsky[xiii] on sleep deprivation and fragmentation found a hyperactivation in host defences and immune mediators, even during catch up sleep, further suggesting that fragmentation of sleep and airway is a potent inducer of MCAS.

Afferent autonomic neurones innervate mast cells, which can degranulate in response to stimulation. While mast cells are viewed more due to their function in allergic reactions, it is now clear that they are important modulators of both nonspecific and specific immune responses. Mast cells are found strategically around capillary beds in connective tissue and on all mucosal surfaces. Their immediate surroundings are rich in autonomic innervation, neuropeptides, and cytokines. Mast cells include prepared cytokines such as TNF-alpha and potentially IL-4, in addition to the more well-known mediators such as histamine[xiv].

These cytokines have strong immunoregulatory effects on lymphocytes and monocytes, affecting the Th1/Th2 balance. Mast cells are therefore prepared to function as cellular transducers of autonomic signals that influence immunological responses. Variations in sleep and wakefulness, which are linked to changes in sympathetic activity, may thereby impact mast cell function and, as a result, mucosal defence responses.

Sleep-deprived rats, for example, may have necrotic skin lesions due to abnormal cytokine release in response to sympathetic nervous system activation of intradermal mast cells, and sleep-induced breakdown in mucosal integrity may be a cause of septicaemia. As we have spoken above the more fragmented the sleep and airway, the more the release of sympathetic chemicals including cortisol and adrenaline.

By this stage I am hopeful you can see the cycle that Mast cells and sleep and airway fragmentation have together. Each can cause or worsen the other.

However, as my premise is that the first dysregulation that occurs is at 5 weeks in utero, creating midline and brainstem dysfunction, retention of primitive reflexes with a greater endpoint of mouth breathing, and that all mouth breathing sets up immune hyperactivation, then I propose that this may be a mechanism that enhances the likely endpoint of MCAS in susceptible patients creating the vast plethora of dysfunctions that is seen in both the OAFMS and MCAS patient. I am certain that patients with OSA and other conditions mentioned in this book are more likely to have MCAS, and that MCAS patients should during history taking during their screening be asked about maternal environment up to 2 years prior to the pregnancy, what the pregnancy was like, and the signs of OAFMS, including mouth breathing, colic, primitive reflex retention, difficulty early on with sleep, tongue and oral fascial restriction, orthodontic work, teeth removal, and so many others as we have previously discussed.

13

To bring this to an End

All diseases are driven by survival compensation as co-ordinated by the brain and include hyperactivation of inflammation as a response to threat, be it hypoxia, low circulation, poor nourishment, lack of connection, or perhaps an inability to communicate effectively with a caregiver. This then becomes expressed by loss of harmony as demonstrated as a ramified immune system, with increase in the release of IL6, TNF-a, CRP, suppression of TGF-b and IL10, and an increased systemic vigilance that pervades neurocognitive development. All of which can be considered as part of an organised survival response.

There are fundamentally 2 states of being, either approach or withdrawal. This is seen in the ANS as rest/digest which is parasympathetic dominant or fight/flight which is considered sympathetic dominant. While this actually acts as a continuum in reality, and that different areas will have different levels of vagal tone, as an organism, one cannot rest/digest and heal when one is fighting for one's life and /or running away.

If the initial threat response that started at 5 weeks gestation is not harmonised to induce neurocognitive inhibition of the primitive reflexes, leading to integration and "normal" development does not ensue, then the child's vigilance set point for survival will be higher than normal, this alters the set point of the nervous system, and can lead to any and all of the disease process's starting that become diagnosed in later life.

This is the Continuum that I have been referring to through the book. It starts early in life and is missed as a significant issue, dismissed even. However, with more chances to catch the continuum and intervene, as it presents to many different practitioners along the path until chronic disease is the result. We are locking our children into a lifetime of health consequences because we don't consider tongue tie important if they can bottle feed and we neglect the importance of airway patency issues in the infant and growing child. We dismiss primitive reflexes to the basket of useless things that are just "grown out of", unimportant, rarely assessed, and when they are, they are either poorly performed or likely misinterpreted to their significance.

We don't connect that orthodontics are not a rite of passage, nor that bruxism is a tool to defend the airway, not just a stress response, both in kids and adults. We paper over so many things from a behavioural psychology point of view that it is harming our society. It is creating unnecessary ill health, both physically and mentally that may very well be unnecessary if we intervened and rehabilitated early and redirected the child's growth trajectory. We spend unnecessarily on medicine, and allied health services because we failed to see the connection between the conditions I spoke about, how posture is affected by both the physical aspects of cranial maldevelopment as well as from breathing issues or retained primitive reflexes, and its capacity to cause breathing issues and effect mood.

We must create a screening program that considers the points raised in this book and start intervening to rehabilitate the young if we want to improve our health outcomes.

The Continuum of ill health has roots that can be traced to the two years prior to mum becoming pregnant, through the gestation and on through life till we are ravaged by infirmity and die earlier than needed.

We need to step back and look at the big picture and follow the indicators to come to the only sensible conclusion, this being that Oral-fascial-cranial maldevelopment causes the three largest threats to human health, that must be arrested and healed.

Those being Sleep fragmentation and airway disruption along with MCAS.

Humans do not fall into discrete diagnosable boxes. Such as Autism type 3, or ADHD with anxiety, or perhaps Obesity and OSA. They almost entirely grew into the condition, it was a journey that had complex issues along the way, physically, neurologically, and biochemically that got them to whichever point on the continuum that you are now assessing, or if as a patient being assessed at.

The journey of how the issue developed is important. It is the continuum that we live in.

May it be a great one for you.

Bibliography

[i] Carol A. Everson, Bernard M. Bergmann, Allan Rechtschaffen, Sleep Deprivation in the Rat: III. Total Sleep Deprivation, *Sleep*, Volume 12, Issue 1, January 1989, Pages 13–21, https://doi.org/10.1093/sleep/12.1.13

[ii] Zachary M. Weil, Greg J. Norman, Kate Karelina, John S. Morris, Jacqueline M. Barker, Alan J. Su, James C. Walton, Steven Bohinc, Randy J. Nelson, A. Courtney DeVries, Sleep deprivation attenuates inflammatory responses and ischemic cell death, Experimental Neurology, Volume 218, Issue 1, 2009, Pages 129-136,

[iii] Mitochondrial oxidative stress after carbon monoxide hypoxia in the rat brain. J Zhang, C A PiantadosiPublished October 1, 1992 J Clin Invest. 1992;90(4):1193-1199. https://doi.org/10.1172/JCI115980.

[iv] Ikonomidou, C., & Kaindl, A. M. (2011). Neuronal Death and Oxidative Stress in the Developing Brain. Antioxidants & Redox Signaling, 14(8), 1535–1550. doi:10.1089/ars.2010.3581

[v] Susanto A, Komara I, Arnov ST. Surgical treatment for Kotlow's class III ankyloglossia: A case report. J Int Oral Health [serial online] 2020 [cited 2022 Dec 11];12:401-5. Available from: https://www.jioh.org/text.asp?2020/12/4/401/292751

[vi] Simpson, J. M. (2001). *Infant stress and sleep deprivation as an aetiological basis for the sudden infant death syndrome.* Early Human Development, 61(1), 1–43. doi:10.1016/s0378-3782(00)00127-4

[vii] Preformed metal crowns for primary and permanent molar teeth: review of the literature Ros C. Randall, PhD, MPhil, BChD .(Pediatr Dent. 2002;24:489-500)

[viii] Relationship between Personality Traits and Cooperation of Adolescent Orthodontic Patients Joaquín Amado; Angela Maria Sierra; Alejandro Gallón; Cristina Álvarez; Tiziano Baccetti, Angle Orthod (2008) 78 (4): 688–691.

[ix] Susanto A, Komara I, Arnov ST. Surgical treatment for Kotlow's class III ankyloglossia: A case report. J Int Oral Health [serial online] 2020 [cited 2022 Dec 11];12:401-5. Available from: https://www.jioh.org/text.asp?2020/12/4/401/292751

[x] Susanto A, Komara I, Arnov ST. Surgical treatment for Kotlow's class III ankyloglossia: A case report. J Int Oral Health [serial online] 2020 [cited 2022 Dec 11];12:401-5. Available from: https://www.jioh.org/text.asp?2020/12/4/401/292751

[xi] Ankyloglossia StatPearls Sarah Becker; Magda D. Mendez. August 22 2022 https://www.ncbi.nlm.nih.gov/books/NBK482295/

[xii] Amitai Y, Shental H, Atkins-Manelis L, Koren G, Zamir CS. Pre-conceptional folic acid supplementation: A possible cause for the increasing rates of ankyloglossia. Med Hypotheses. 2020 Jan;134:109508. doi: 10.1016/j.mehy.2019.109508. Epub 2019 Nov 18. PMID: 31835174.

[xiii] Mills N, Pransky SM, Geddes DT, Mirjalili SA. What is a tongue tie? Defining the anatomy of the in-situ lingual frenulum. Clin Anat. 2019 Sep;32(6):749-761. doi: 10.1002/ca.23343. Epub 2019 Feb 19. PMID: 30701608; PMCID: PMC6850428.

[xiv] Tuchman, D.N. Dysfunctional swallowing in the pediatric patient: Clinical considerations. *Dysphagia* **2**, 203–208 (1988). https://doi.org/10.1007/BF02414427

[xv] Posture and Functional Action in Infancy: Philippe Rochat and André Bullinger, https://www.taylorfrancis.com/books/mono/10.4324/9780203772942/early-child-development-french-tradition?refId=622dd760-175f-4b01-95bf-c186a552ee4a&context=ubx

[xvi] Stein, B.E., Stanford, T.R., Godwin, D.W., McHaffie, J.G. (2013). The Superior Colliculus and Visual Thalamus. In: Pfaff, D.W. (eds) Neuroscience in the 21st Century. Springer, New York, NY. https://doi.org/10.1007/978-1-4614-1997-6_23

[xvii] Isa T, Hall WC. Exploring the superior colliculus in vitro. J Neurophysiol. 2009 Nov;102(5):2581-93. doi: 10.1152/jn.00498.2009. Epub 2009 Aug 26. PMID: 19710376; PMCID: PMC2777828.

[xviii] Porges SW. Vagal tone: a physiologic marker of stress vulnerability. Pediatrics. 1992 Sep;90(3 Pt 2):498-504. PMID: 1513615.

[xix] Infant Behav Dev. 2008 Sep; 31(3): 361–373. Vagal activity, early growth and emotional development Fields T , Diego M

[xx] Killing Me Softly: The Fetal Origins Hypothesis* J Econ Perspect. 2011 ; 25(3): 153–172. doi:10.1257/jep.25.3.153. Douglas Almond and Janet Currie

[xxi] Tuchman, D.N. Dysfunctional swallowing in the pediatric patient: Clinical considerations. Dysphagia 2, 203–208 (1988). https://doi.org/10.1007/BF02414427

[xxii] Tuchman, D.N. Dysfunctional swallowing in the pediatric patient: Clinical considerations. Dysphagia 2, 203–208 (1988). https://doi.org/10.1007/BF02414427

[xxiii] Neuropsychologia 46 (2008) 2851–2854 Mirror neuron activation is associated with facial emotion processing Peter G. Enticott et al

[xxiv] Dev Neurobiol. 2016 Jan; 76(1): 75–92. Zebrafish cerebrospinal fluid mediates cell survival through a retinoid signaling pathway Jessica T. Chang, Maria K. Lehtinen, Hazel Sive

[xxv] Dev Neurobiol. 2016 Jan; 76(1): 75–92. Zebrafish cerebrospinal fluid

mediates cell survival through a retinoid signaling pathway Jessica T. Chang, Maria K. Lehtinen, Hazel Sive

[xxvi] H. Herschel Conaway, Petra Henning, Ulf H. Lerner, Vitamin A Metabolism, Action, and Role in Skeletal Homeostasis, Endocrine Reviews, Volume 34, Issue 6, 1 December 2013, Pages 766–797,

[xxvii] Allyson E. Kennedy, Amanda J.G. Dickinson, Median facial clefts in Xenopus laevis: Roles of retinoic acid signaling and homeobox genes, Developmental Biology, Volume 365, Issue 1,2012, Pages 229-240, ISSN 0012-1606

[xxviii] Wahl, S.E., et al., The role of folate metabolism in orofacial development and clefting. Dev. Biol. (2015),

[xxix] Amitai Y, Shental H, Atkins-Manelis L, Koren G, Zamir CS. Pre-conceptional folic acid supplementation: A possible cause for the increasing rates of ankyloglossia. Med Hypotheses. 2020 Jan;134:109508. doi: 10.1016/j.mehy.2019.109508. Epub 2019 Nov 18. PMID: 31835174.

[xxx] Wan, L., Li, Y., Zhang, Z. et al. Methylenetetrahydrofolate reductase and psychiatric diseases. Transl Psychiatry 8, 242 (2018). https://doi.org/10.1038/s41398-018-0276-6

[xxxi] Amitai Y, Shental H, Atkins-Manelis L, Koren G, Zamir CS. Pre-conceptional folic acid supplementation: A possible cause for the increasing rates of ankyloglossia. Med Hypotheses. 2020 Jan;134:109508. doi: 10.1016/j.mehy.2019.109508. Epub 2019 Nov 18. PMID: 31835174

[xxxii] Wahl, S.E., et al., The role of folate metabolism in orofacial development and clefting. Dev. Biol. (2015),

[xxxiii] Wahl, S.E., et al., The role of folate metabolism in orofacial development and clefting. Dev. Biol. (2015),

[xxxiv] Brooklyin S, Jana R, Aravinthan S, Adhisivam B, Chand P. Assessment of Folic Acid and DNA Damage in Cleft Lip and Cleft Palate. Clinics and Practice. 2014; 4(1):608. https://doi.org/10.4081/cp.2014.608

[xxxv] Wahl, S.E., et al., The role of folate metabolism in orofacial development and clefting. Dev. Biol. (2015),

[xxxvi] FACIAL AND PALATAL DEVELOPMENT Letty Moss-Salentijn DDS, PhD, Dr. Edwin S.Robinson Professor of Dentistry (in Anatomy and Cell Biology) E-mail: lm23@columbia.edu Chapter 11.

[xxxvii] Ferguson, J., & Atit, R. P. (2018). A tale of two cities: the genetic mechanisms governing calvarial bone development. Genesis. doi:10.1002/dvg.23248

[xxxviii] Yuji Mishina, Taylor Nicholas Snider, Neural crest cell signaling pathways critical to cranial bone development and pathology, Experimental Cell Research, Volume 325, Issue 2, 2014, Pages 138-147

[xxxix] Dickinson AJG, Turner SD, Wahl S, Kennedy AE, Wyatt BH, Howton DA. E-liquids and vanillin flavoring disrupts retinoic acid signaling and causes

craniofacial defects in Xenopus embryos. Dev Biol. 2022 Jan;481:14-29. doi: 10.1016/j.ydbio.2021.09.004. Epub 2021 Sep 17. PMID: 34543654; PMCID: PMC8665092.

[xl] Australian Bureau of Statistics (December 2011), Australian Health Survey: Biomedical Results for Nutrients, ABS Website, accessed 12 December 2022.

[xli] Australian Bureau of Statistics (December 2011), Australian Health Survey: Biomedical Results for Nutrients, ABS Website, accessed 12 December 2022.

[xlii] Messner AH, Lalakea ML, Aby J, Macmahon J, Bair E. Ankyloglossia: Incidence and Associated Feeding Difficulties. Arch Otolaryngol Head Neck Surg. 2000;126(1):36–39. doi:10.1001/archotol.126.1.36

[xliii] De Ridder L, Aleksieva A, Willems G, Declerck D, Cadenas de Llano-Pérula M. Prevalence of Orthodontic Malocclusions in Healthy Children and Adolescents: A Systematic Review. Int J Environ Res Public Health. 2022 Jun 17;19(12):7446. doi: 10.3390/ijerph19127446. PMID: 35742703; PMCID: PMC9223594.

[xliv] Lizal F, Elcner J, Jedelsky J, Maly M, Jicha M, Farkas Á, Belka M, Rehak Z, Adam J, Brinek A, Laznovsky J, Zikmund T, Kaiser J. The effect of oral and nasal breathing on the deposition of inhaled particles in upper and tracheobronchial airways. J Aerosol Sci. 2020 Dec;150:105649. doi: 10.1016/j.jaerosci.2020.105649. Epub 2020 Aug 28. PMID: 32904428; PMCID: PMC7455204.

[xlv] Paediatrics and Child Health Division of The Royal Australasian College of Physicians and The Australian Society of Otolaryngology, Head and Neck Surgery. 2008. Indications for tonsillectomy and adenotonsillectomy in children: A joint position paper.

[xlvi] Georgalas CC, Tolley NS, Narula PA. Tonsillitis. BMJ Clin Evid. 2014 Jul 22;2014:0503. PMID: 25051184; PMCID: PMC4106232.

[xlvii] Tsung-Hsueh Hsieh, Po-Yen Chen, Fang-Liang Huang, Jiann-Der Wang, Li-Ching Wang, Heng-Kuei Lin, Hsiao-Chuan Lin, Hsin-Yang Hsieh, Meng-Kung Yu, Chih-Feng Chang, Tzu-Yau Chuang, Chin-Yun Lee, Are empiric antibiotics for acute exudative tonsillitis needed in children?, Journal of Microbiology, Immunology and Infection, Volume 44, Issue 5, 2011, Pages 328-332,

[xlviii] Hoffman Kevin W., Lee Jakleen J., Corcoran Cheryl M., Kimhy David, Kranz Thorsten M., Malaspina Dolores Considering the Microbiome in Stress-Related and Neurodevelopmental Trajectories to Schizophrenia Frontiers in Psychiatry VOLUME 11 2020

[xlix] Blaser, M. J. (2016). Antibiotic use and its consequences for the normal microbiome. Science, 352(6285), 544–545. doi:10.1126/science.aad9358

Bibliography • 255

[l] Blaser, M. J. (2016). Antibiotic use and its consequences for the normal microbiome. Science, 352(6285), 544–545. doi:10.1126/science.aad9358

[li] Solow, B., Ovesen, J., Nielsen, P. W., Wildschiodtz, G., & Tallgren, A. (1993). Head posture in obstructive sleep apnoea. European Orthodontic Society, 15, 107–114.

[lii] Meiyappan, N., Tamizharasi, S., Senthilkumar, K. P., & Janardhanan, K. (2015). Natural Head Position: An Overview. Journal of Pharmacy and BioAllied Sciences, August(Suppl 2), S424–S427.

[liii] Uhlig, S. E., Marchesi, L. M., Duarte, H., & Araújo, M. T. M. (2015). Association between respiratory and postural adaptations and self-perception of school-aged children with mouth breathing in relation to their quality of life. Brazilian Journal of Physical Therapy, 19(3), 201–210.

[liv] Implications of mouth breathing on the pulmonary function and respiratory muscles Helenize Lopes Veron(1) Ana Gabrieli Antunes(1) Jovana de Moura Milanesi(1) Eliane Castilhos Rodrigues Corrêa(2) Rev. CEFAC. 2016 Jan-Fev; 18(1):242-251 doi: 10.1590/1982-0216201618111915

[lv] Yeol, H., Jong, K., Jeong, I., Jung, H. D., Sohn, H., Duk, S., … Yun, S. (2013). Nasal Obstruction and Palate-Tongue Position on Sleep-Disordered Breathing. Clinical and Experimental Otohinolaryngology, 6(4), 226–230.

[lvi] Uhlig, S. E., Marchesi, L. M., Duarte, H., & Araújo, M. T. M. (2015). Association between respiratory and postural adaptations and self-perception of school-aged children with mouth breathing in relation to their quality of life. Brazilian Journal of Physical Therapy, 19(3), 201–210.

[lvii] Implications of mouth breathing on the pulmonary function and respiratory muscles Helenize Lopes Veron(1) Ana Gabrieli Antunes(1) Jovana de Moura Milanesi(1) Eliane Castilhos Rodrigues Corrêa(2) Rev. CEFAC. 2016 Jan-Fev; 18(1):242-251 doi: 10.1590/1982-0216201618111915

[lviii] Rengasamy Venugopalan S, Van Otterloo E. The Skull's Girder: A Brief Review of the Cranial Base. J Dev Biol. 2021 Jan 23;9(1):3. doi: 10.3390/jdb9010003. PMID: 33498686; PMCID: PMC7838769.

[lix] HINCK VC, HOPKINS CE. Concerning Growth of the Sphenoid Sinus. Arch Otolaryngol. 1965;82(1):62–66. doi:10.1001/archotol.1965.00760010064015

[lx] http://www.columbia.edu/itc/hs/medical/humandev/2004/Chapt11-FacialPalatalDev.pdf

[lxi] Jain P, Rathee M. Embryology, Tongue. [Updated 2022 Aug 8]. In: StatPearls [Internet]. Treasure Island (FL): StatPearls Publishing; 2022 Jan-. Available from: https://www.ncbi.nlm.nih.gov/books/NBK547697/

[lxii] Maloclusion and its far reaching Effects Samuel Adams Cohen Journal American Medical Association 1922 Vol 79, number 23 pg 1895-1897

[lxiii] Maloclusion and its far reaching Effects Samuel Adams Cohen Journal American Medical Association 1922 Vol 79, number 23 pg 1895-1897

[lxiv] Breathe, Sleep, Thrive: Discover how airway health can unlock your child's greater health, learning, and potential Lim, Shereen Published by Sparkle Publishing, 2022 ISBN 10: 0645553212ISBN 13: 9780645553215

[lxv] Tuchman, D.N. Dysfunctional swallowing in the pediatric patient: Clinical considerations. Dysphagia 2, 203–208 (1988). https://doi.org/10.1007/BF02414427

[lxvi] Yamaguchi H, Tada S, Nakanishi Y, Kawaminami S, Shin T, Tabata R, Yuasa S, Shimizu N, Kohno M, Tsuchiya A, Tani K. Association between Mouth Breathing and Atopic Dermatitis in Japanese Children 2-6 years Old: A Population-Based Cross-Sectional Study. PLoS One. 2015 Apr 27;10(4):e0125916. doi: 10.1371/journal.pone.0125916. PMID: 25915864; PMCID: PMC4411141.

[lxvii] https://www.rch.org.au/clinicalguide/guideline_index/Gastrooesophageal_reflux_disease_in_infants/

[lxviii] Justiz Vaillant AA, Modi P, Jan A. Atopy. [Updated 2022 Jul 8]. In: StatPearls [Internet]. Treasure Island (FL): StatPearls Publishing; 2022 Jan-. Available from: https://www.ncbi.nlm.nih.gov/books/NBK542187/

[lxix] Lee DW, Kim JG, Yang YM. Influence of mouth breathing on atopic dermatitis risk and oral health in children: A population-based cross-sectional study. J Dent Sci. 2021 Jan;16(1):178-185. doi: 10.1016/j.jds.2020.06.014. Epub 2020 Jun 22. PMID: 33384795; PMCID: PMC7770290.

[lxx] https://birthinjurycenter.org/causes-of-infant-brain-injuries/

[lxxi] https://www.aihw.gov.au/reports/mothers-babies/australias-mothers-babies/contents/labour-and-birth/method-of-birth

[lxxii] https://www.abs.gov.au/statistics/people/population/births-australia/latest-release

[lxxiii] Linda J. Smith, Impact of Birthing Practices on the Breastfeeding Dyad, Journal of Midwifery & Women's Health, Volume 52, Issue 6, 2007,Pages 621-630,

[lxxiv] Robert T. Hall, Anne M. Mercer, Susan L. Teasley, Deanna M. McPherson, Stephen D. Simon, Susan R. Santos, Bridget M. Meyers, Nancy E. Hipsh, A breast-feeding assessment score to evaluate the risk for cessation of breast-feeding by 7 to 10 days of age, The Journal of Pediatrics, Volume 141, Issue 5,2002

[lxxv] Posture and Functional Action in Infancy: Philippe Rochat and André Bullinger, https://www.taylorfrancis.com/books/mono/10.4324/9780203772942/early-child-development-french-tradition?refId=622dd760-175f-4b01-95bf-c186a552ee4a&context=ubx

[lxxvi] Luers JC, Hüttenbrink KB. Surgical anatomy and pathology of the middle ear. J Anat. 2016 Feb;228(2):338-53. doi: 10.1111/joa.12389. Epub 2015 Oct 19. PMID: 26482007; PMCID: PMC4718166.

Bibliography • 257

[lxxvii] Exar EN, Collop NA. The upper airway resistance syndrome. Chest. 1999 Apr;115(4):1127-39. doi: 10.1378/chest.115.4.1127. PMID: 10208219.

[lxxviii] Tanaka T, Narazaki M, Kishimoto T. IL-6 in inflammation, immunity, and disease. Cold Spring Harb Perspect Biol. 2014 Sep 4;6(10):a016295. doi: 10.1101/cshperspect.a016295. PMID: 25190079; PMCID: PMC4176007.

[lxxix] Kim, J., Bhattacharjee, R., Dayyat, E. et al. Increased Cellular Proliferation and Inflammatory Cytokines in Tonsils Derived From Children With Obstructive Sleep Apnea. Pediatr Res 66, 423–428 (2009). https://doi.org/10.1203/PDR.0b013e3181b453e3

[lxxx] Mosaad Abdel-Aziz, Neamat Ibrahim, Abeer Ahmed, Mostafa El-Hamamsy, Mohamed I. Abdel-Khalik, Hassan El-Hoshy, Lingual tonsils hypertrophy; a cause of obstructive sleep apnea in children after adenotonsillectomy: Operative problems and management, International Journal of Pediatric Otorhinolaryngology, Volume 75, Issue 9, 2011, Pages 1127-1131,

[lxxxi] Paediatrics and Child Health Division of The Royal Australasian College of Physicians and The Australian Society of Otolaryngology, Head and Neck Surgery. 2008. Indications for tonsillectomy and adenotonsillectomy in children: A joint position paper.

[lxxxii] Harvold E. P., Tomer B. S., Vargervik K., Chierici G. (1981). Primate experiments on oral respiration. Am. J. Orthod. 79, 359–372 10.1016/0002-9416(81)90379-1

[lxxxiii] Vargervik K., Miller A. J., Chierici G., Harvold E., Tomer B. S. (1984). Morphologic response to changes in neuromuscular patterns experimentally induced by altered modes of respiration. Am. J. Orthod. 85, 115–124

[lxxxiv] Miller A. J., Vargervik K., Chierici G. (1984). Experimentally induced neuromuscular changes during and after nasal airway obstruction. Am. J. Orthod. 85, 385–392 10.1016/0002-9416(84)90159-3

[lxxxv] Miller AJ, Vargervik K, Chierici G. Experimentally induced neuromuscular changes during and after nasal airway obstruction. Am J Orthod. 1984 May;85(5):385-92. doi: 10.1016/0002-9416(84)90159-3. PMID: 6586077.

[lxxxvi] Diagnosis and Treatment of ADHD in the United States: Update by Gender and Race, Kathleen A. Fairman1 , Alyssa M. Peckham1 , and David A. Sclar, Journal of Attention Disorders 2020, Vol. 24(1) 10–19

[lxxxvii] Rethinking ADHD: From brain to Culture, By Sami Timimi, Jonathan Leo Red Globe Press; First edition (March 31, 2009).

[lxxxviii] Ehrlich PR, Levin SA.. 2005. The evolution of norms. Public Library of Science 3: 943–948.

[lxxxix] Christopherson EA, Briskie D, Inglehart MR. 2009. Objective, subjective, and self-assessment of preadolescent orthodontic treatment need: A function

of age, gender, and ethnic/racial background? Journal of Public Health Dentistry 69: 9–17.

[xc] Vgontzas, A., & Pavlović, J. M. (2018). Sleep Disorders and Migraine: Review of Literature and Potential Pathophysiology Mechanisms. Headache: The Journal of Head and Face Pain.

[xci] Vgontzas, A., & Pavlović, J. M. (2018). Sleep Disorders and Migraine: Review of Literature and Potential Pathophysiology Mechanisms. Headache: The Journal of Head and Face Pain.

[xci] Onen, S. H., Onen, F., Courpron, P., & Dubray, C. (2005). How Pain and Analgesics Disturb Sleep. The Clinical Journal of Pain, 21(5), 422–431. doi:10.1097/01.ajp.0000129757.

[xcii] Onen, S. H., Onen, F., Courpron, P., & Dubray, C. (2005). How Pain and Analgesics Disturb Sleep. The Clinical Journal of Pain, 21(5), 422–431. doi:10.1097/01.ajp.0000129757.

[xciii] Vgontzas, A., & Pavlović, J. M. (2018). Sleep Disorders and Migraine: Review of Literature and Potential Pathophysiology Mechanisms. Headache: The Journal of Head and Face Pain.

[xciv] Da Vitoria Lobo, Marlene E.a; Weir, Nickb; Hardowar, Lydiab; Al Ojaimi, Yarab; Madden, Ryana; Gibson, Alexa; Bestall, Samuel M.c; Hirashima, Masanorid; Schaffer, Chris B.e; Donaldson, Lucy F.c; Bates, David O.a,f; Hulse, Richard Philipa,b,*. Hypoxia-induced carbonic anhydrase mediated dorsal horn neuron activation and induction of neuropathic pain. PAIN 163(11):p 2264-2279, November 2022

[xcv] Guilleminault C, De Los Reyes V. 2011. Upper-airway resistance syndrome. Handbook of Clinical Neurology 98: 401–409.

[xcvi] Journal of Aesthetic NursingVol. 11, No. 4Clinical Dynamic muscle discord in the context of non-surgical lip enhancement Dean Rhobaye Published Online:2 May 2022https://doi.org/10.12968/joan.2022.11.4.174

[xcvii] Modrell AK, Tadi P. Primitive Reflexes. [Updated 2022 Mar 9]. In: StatPearls [Internet]. Treasure Island (FL): StatPearls Publishing; 2022 Jan-. Available from: https://www.ncbi.nlm.nih.gov/books/NBK554606/

[xcviii] Porges SW (2011). The Polyvagal Theory: Neurophysiological Foundations of Emotions, Attachment, Communication, and Self-regulation. New York: WW Norton.

[xcix] Breit Sigrid, Kupferberg Aleksandra, Rogler Gerhard, Hasler Gregor Vagus Nerve as Modulator of the Brain–Gut Axis in Psychiatric and Inflammatory Disorders Frontiers in Psychiatry VOLUME 9, 2018 https://www.frontiersin.org/articles/10.3389/fpsyt.2018.00044

[c] Simpson, J. M. (2001). Infant stress and sleep deprivation as an aetiological basis for the sudden infant death syndrome. Early Human Development, 61(1), 1–43. doi:10.1016/s0378-3782(00)00127-4

[ci] Becker LE, Zhang W, Pereyra PM. Delayed maturation of the vagus nerve in

sudden infant death syndrome. Acta Neuropathol. 1993;86(6):617-22. doi: 10.1007/BF00294301. PMID: 8310817.

[cii] Birger Kaada, The sudden infant death syndrome induced by 'the fear paralysis reflex', Medical Hypotheses, Volume 22, Issue 4, 1987, Pages 347-356, ISSN 0306-9877,

[ciii] Becker LE, Zhang W, Pereyra PM. Delayed maturation of the vagus nerve in sudden infant death syndrome. Acta Neuropathol. 1993;86(6):617-22. doi: 10.1007/BF00294301. PMID: 8310817

[civ] Bednarczuk N, Milner A, Greenough A. The Role of Maternal Smoking in Sudden Fetal and Infant Death Pathogenesis. Front Neurol. 2020 Oct 23;11:586068. doi: 10.3389/fneur.2020.586068. PMID: 33193050; PMCID: PMC7644853.

[cv] Kaada B. The sudden infant death syndrome induced by "the fear paralysis reflex'? Med Hypotheses. 1987 Apr;22(4):347-56. doi: 10.1016/0306-9877(87)90029-6. PMID: 3647223.

[cvi] Hajdusianek W, Żórawik A, Waliszewska-Prosół M, Poręba R, Gać P. Tobacco and Nervous System Development and Function-New Findings 2015-2020. Brain Sci. 2021 Jun 16;11(6):797. doi: 10.3390/brainsci11060797. PMID: 34208753; PMCID: PMC8234722.

[cvii] The origin of REM sleep: A hypothesis. Tsoukalas, I. (2012). The origin of REM sleep: A hypothesis. Dreaming, 22(4), 253–283. https://doi.org/10.1037/a0030790

[cviii] Control of Upper Airway Motoneurons During REM Sleep
Leszek Kubin, Richard O. Davies, and Allan I. Pack
01 APR 1998https://doi.org/10.1152/physiologyonline.1998.13.2.91

[cix] Spencer AE, Marin MF, Milad MR, Spencer TJ, Bogucki OE, Pope AL, Plasencia N, Hughes B, Pace-Schott EF, Fitzgerald M, Uchida M, Biederman J. Abnormal fear circuitry in Attention Deficit Hyperactivity Disorder: A controlled magnetic resonance imaging study. Psychiatry Res Neuroimaging. 2017 Apr 30;262:55-62. doi: 10.1016/j.pscychresns.2016.12.015. Epub 2017 Feb 10. PMID: 28235692.

[cx] Norcliffe-Kaufmann L, Palma JA, Martinez J, Camargo C, Kaufmann H. Fear conditioning as a pathogenic mechanism in the postural tachycardia syndrome. Brain. 2022 Nov 21;145(11):3763-3769. doi: 10.1093/brain/awac249. PMID: 35802513.

[cxi] Rousseau, P. V., Matton, F., Lecuyer, R., & Lahaye, W. (2017). The Moro reaction: More than a reflex, a ritualized behavior of nonverbal communication. Infant Behavior and Development, 46, 169–177. doi:10.1016/j.infbeh.2017.01.004

[cxii] Rousseau, P. V., Matton, F., Lecuyer, R., & Lahaye, W. (2017). The Moro reaction: More than a reflex, a ritualized behavior of nonverbal communication. Infant Behavior and Development, 46, 169–177.

doi:10.1016/j.infbeh.2017.01.0

[cxiii] Lau C. Development of Suck and Swallow Mechanisms in Infants. Ann Nutr Metab. 2015;66 Suppl 5(0 5):7-14. doi: 10.1159/000381361. Epub 2015 Jul 24. PMID: 26226992; PMCID: PMC4530609.

[cxiv] Rousseau, P. V., Matton, F., Lecuyer, R., & Lahaye, W. (2017). The Moro reaction: More than a reflex, a ritualized behavior of nonverbal communication. Infant Behavior and Development, 46, 169–177. doi:10.1016/j.infbeh.2017.01.0

[cxv] Prevalence of primitive reflexes and or frontal release sign in the substance abuse populations Oeyvind Andreassen1*, Sverre M. Nesvåg2 and Anne-Lill M. Nja2 1 Salvation Army Treatment Center Stavanger (FAB), FAB, Norway 2 Regionalt kompetansesenter for rusmiddelforskning i Helse Vest, KORFOR, Norway

[cxvi] Gieysztor EZ, Choińska AM, Paprocka-Borowicz M. Persistence of primitive reflexes and associated motor problems in healthy preschool children. Arch Med Sci. 2018 Jan;14(1):167-173. doi: 10.5114/aoms.2016.60503. Epub 2016 Jun 13. PMID: 29379547; PMCID: PMC5778413.

[cxvii] Gieysztor EZ, Choińska AM, Paprocka-Borowicz M. Persistence of primitive reflexes and associated motor problems in healthy preschool children. Arch Med Sci. 2018 Jan;14(1):167-173. doi: 10.5114/aoms.2016.60503. Epub 2016 Jun 13. PMID: 29379547; PMCID: PMC5778413.

[cxviii] The Correlation between Primitive Reflexes and Saccadic Eye Movements in 5th Grade Children with Teacher-Reported Reading Problems. Source: Optometry & Vision Development . 2008, Vol. 39 Issue 3, p140-145. 6p. Author(s): González, Sergio Ramírez; Ciuffreda, Kenneth J.; Hernández, Luís Castillo; Escalante, Jaime Bernal

[cxix] Pierre V. Rousseau, Florence Matton, Renaud Lecuyer, Willy Lahaye, The Moro reaction: More than a reflex, a ritualized behavior of nonverbal communication, Infant Behavior and Development, Volume 46,2017, Pages 169-177,

[cxx] CURRENT LITERATURE; II. SENSORI-MOTOR NEUROLOGY; 3. SPINAL CORD.: PDF ONLY
SPINAL REFLEX Galant, S.The Journal OF Nervous and Mental Disease 51(5):p 496, May 1920.

[cxxi] Desorbay T. A neuro-developmental approach to specific learning difficulties. Int J Nutr Pharmacol Neurol Dis 2013;3:1-2

[cxxii] PERSISTENCE OF PRIMITIVE REFLEXES AND ASSOCIATED PROBLEMS IN CHILDREN Olivera RASHIKJ-CANEVSKA UDK: 159.922-053.2 Monika MIHAJLOVSKA December 2019 DOI: 10.37510/godzbo1972513rc

[cxxiii] Konicarova, J., Bob, P. Retained Primitive Reflexes and ADHD in

Children. Act Nerv Super54, 135–138 (2012). https://doi.org/10.1007/BF03379591
[cxxiv] Neurophysiological Foundation of the MNRI® Reflex Integration Program S. Masgutova, Ph.D, USA; Denis Masgutov, ISMI Director & Program Co-Creator, Poland; Nelli Akhmatova, MD, Ph.D, Russia; Elvin Akhmatov, MA., Ph.D Student, USA 2015, Svetlana Masgutova Educational Institute® for Neuro-Sensory-Motor and Reflex Integration, SMEI (USA)
[cxxv] VOLLMER H. A New Reflex in Young Infants. AMA Am J Dis Child. 1958;95(5):481–484. doi:10.1001/archpedi.1958.02060050485004
[cxxvi] Powerful! Reflexes help shape your life. Barbel Holscher 2014
[cxxvii] Powerful! Reflexes help shape your life. Barbel Holscher 2014
[cxxviii] Powerful! Reflexes help shape your life. Barbel Holscher 2014
[cxxix] Griffioen, M., van Drunen, P., Maaswinkel, E. et al. Identification of intrinsic and reflexive contributions to trunk stabilization in patients with low back pain: a case–control study.Eur Spine J 29, 1900–1908 (2020). https://doi.org/10.1007/s00586-020-06385-9
[cxxx] Developmental Gains for a Child With Dyslexia and Allergies
Beata Oginska-Dutkiewicz, MA, and Teresa-Ewa Busz, MA, MNRI® Core Specialists and Instructors, Zielona Gora, Poland 2015, Svetlana Masgutova Educational Institute® for Neuro-Sensory-Motor and Reflex Integration, SMEI (USA)
[cxxxi] Powerful! Reflexes help shape your life. Barbel Holscher 2014 Book
[cxxxii] Van Gijn J The Babinski reflex. Postgraduate Medical Journal 1995;71:645-648.
[cxxxiii] Van Gijn J The Babinski reflex. Postgraduate Medical Journal 1995;71:645-648.
[cxxxiv] Arcilla CK, Vilella RC. Tonic Neck Reflex. [Updated 2022 May 8]. In: StatPearls [Internet]. Treasure Island (FL): StatPearls Publishing; 2022 Jan-. Available from: https://www.ncbi.nlm.nih.gov/books/NBK559210/
[cxxxv] Arcilla CK, Vilella RC. Tonic Neck Reflex. [Updated 2022 May 8]. In: StatPearls [Internet]. Treasure Island (FL): StatPearls Publishing; 2022 Jan-. Available from: https://www.ncbi.nlm.nih.gov/books/NBK559210/
[cxxxvi] The Primitive Reflexes: Considerations in the Infant. Optometry & Vision Development . 2006, Vol. 37 Issue 3, p139-145. 8p. Berne, Samuel A.
[cxxxvii] Diana R. Feldhacker, Reilly Cosgrove, Ben Feiten, Kayleigh Schmidt & Marissa Stewart (2022) The Correlation between Retained Primitive Reflexes and Scholastic Performance among Early Elementary Students, Journal of Occupational Therapy, Schools, & Early Intervention, 15:3, 288-301
[cxxxviii] Martin McPhillips, Julie-Anne Jordan-Black, Primary reflex persistence in children with reading difficulties (dyslexia): A cross-sectional study, Neuropsychologia, Volume 45, Issue 4, 2007, Pages 748-754, ISSN 0028-3932,
[cxxxix] Martin McPhillips, Julie-Anne Jordan-Black, Primary reflex persistence in

children with reading difficulties (dyslexia): A cross-sectional study, Neuropsychologia, Volume 45, Issue 4, 2007, Pages 748-754, ISSN 0028-3932

[cxl] The Rhythmic Movement Method: A Revolutionary Approach to Improved Health and Well-Being Author Harald Blomberg, MD ISBN 1483428796, 9781483428796

[cxli] The Correlation between Primitive Reflexes and Saccadic Eye Movements in 5th Grade Children with Teacher-Reported Reading Problems. Optometry & Vision Development . 2008, Vol. 39 Issue 3, p140-145. 6p. González, Sergio Ramírez; Ciuffreda, Kenneth J.; Hernández, Luís Castillo; Escalante, Jaime Bernal

[cxlii] Andrich P, Shihada MB, Vinci MK, Wrenhaven SL, Goodman GG. Statistical Relationships Between Visual Skill Deficits and Retained Primitive Reflexes in Children. Optom Vis Perf 2018;6(3):106-11.

[cxliii] Diana R. Feldhacker, Reilly Cosgrove, Ben Feiten, Kayleigh Schmidt & Marissa Stewart (2022) The Correlation between Retained Primitive Reflexes and Scholastic Performance among Early Elementary Students, Journal of Occupational Therapy, Schools, & Early Intervention, 15:3, 288-301

[cxliv] Arcilla CK, Vilella RC. Tonic Neck Reflex. [Updated 2022 May 8]. In: StatPearls [Internet]. Treasure Island (FL): StatPearls Publishing; 2022 Jan-. Available from: https://www.ncbi.nlm.nih.gov/books/NBK559210/

[cxlv] Connolly BH, Michael BT. Early detection of scoliosis. A neurological approach using the asymmetrical tonic neck reflex. Phys Ther. 1984 Mar;64(3):304-7. doi: 10.1093/ptj/64.3.304. PMID: 6701200.

[cxlvi] Affective Neuroscience, The foundations of Human And Animal Emotions. Jaak Panskeep. 1998 Oxford university Press

[cxlvii] The Landau Reaction (Reflex) Ross G mitchell Developmental Medicine and Child Neurology Volume4, Issue1 February 1962 Pages 65-70

[cxlviii] Powerful! Reflexes help shape your life. Barbel Holscher 2014

[cxlix] Somatics: Reawakening The Mind's Control Of Movement, Flexibility, And Health Thomas Hanna

[cl] S.M. Bruijn, F. Massaad, M.J. MacLellan, L. Van Gestel, Y.P. Ivanenko, J. Duysens, Are effects of the symmetric and asymmetric tonic neck reflexes still visible in healthy adults?, Neuroscience Letters, Volume 556,2013,Pages 89-92,

[cli] Blum CL. R + C Factors and Sacro Occipital Technique Orthopedic Blocking: a pilot study using pre and post VAS assessment. J Can Chiropr Assoc. 2015 Jun;59(2):134-42. PMID: 26136605; PMCID: PMC4486986.

[clii] Blum CL. R + C Factors and Sacro Occipital Technique Orthopedic Blocking: a pilot study using pre and post VAS assessment. J Can Chiropr Assoc. 2015 Jun;59(2):134-42. PMID: 26136605; PMCID: PMC4486986.

[cliii] Gatt A, Agarwal S, Zito PM. Anatomy, Fascia Layers. [Updated 2022 Jul 25]. In: StatPearls [Internet]. Treasure Island (FL): StatPearls Publishing; 2022 Jan-.

[cliv] Encyclopedia of Respiratory Medicine. (2006) ISBN: 9780123708793
[clv] Anthony Henry Vernon Schapira, Edward Byrne (M.D.). Neurology and Clinical Neuroscience. (2007) ISBN: 9780323033541
[clvi] The Master and His Emissary: The Divided Brain and the Making of the Western World Paperback – Illustrated, 14 February 2019
[clvii] Shandley Sabrina, Capilouto Gilson, Tamilia Eleonora, Riley David M., Johnson Yvette R., Papadelis Christos Abnormal Nutritive Sucking as an Indicator of Neonatal Brain Injury Frontiers in Pediatrics VOLUME 8, 2021
[clviii] Kaur, Charanpreet & Mukesh, Chandra & Sharma, Mukesh. (2016). A Study to Assess the Sucking Reflex of Neonates Born at Selected Hospitals. International Journal of Science and Research (IJSR). 5. 6-391.
[clix] Shandley Sabrina, Capilouto Gilson, Tamilia Eleonora, Riley David M., Johnson Yvette R., Papadelis Christo. Abnormal Nutritive Sucking as an Indicator of Neonatal Brain Injury Frontiers in Pediatrics VOLUME 8, 2021 DOI=10.3389/fped.2020.599633
[clx] Yoo H, Mihaila DM. Rooting Reflex. [Updated 2022 Apr 28]. In: StatPearls [Internet]. Treasure Island (FL): StatPearls Publishing; 2022 Jan-. Available from: https://www.ncbi.nlm.nih.gov/books/NBK557636/
[clxi] Walker HK. The Suck, Snout, Palmomental, and Grasp Reflexes. In: Walker HK, Hall WD, Hurst JW, editors. Clinical Methods: The History, Physical, and Laboratory Examinations. 3rd edition. Boston: Butterworths; 1990. Chapter 71. Available from: https://www.ncbi.nlm.nih.gov/books/NBK395/
[clxii] Glabellar Reflex R.C. Shah, in Encyclopedia of Movement Disorders, 2010
[clxiii] Glabellar Reflex R.C. Shah, in Encyclopedia of Movement Disorders, 2010
[clxiv] Mbata G, Chukwuka J. Obstructive sleep apnea hypopnea syndrome. Ann Med Health Sci Res. 2012 Jan;2(1):74-7. doi: 10.4103/2141-9248.96943. PMID: 23209996; PMCID: PMC3507119.
[clxv] Obstructive Sleep Apnea Patrick J. Strollo, Jr., M.D., and Robert M. Rogers, M.D. N Engl J Med 1996; 334:99-104
[clxvi] REM-related obstructive sleep apnea: when does it matter? Effect on motor memory consolidation versus emotional health Ina Djonlagic, MD; Meng Guo, MD; Moroke Igue, BS; Atul Malhotra, MD; Robert Stickgold, PhD Journal of Clinical Sleep Medicine, Vol. 16, No. 3March 15, 2020377https://doi.org/10.5664/jcsm.8210
[clxvii] Hammond, E. C., & Garfinkel, L. (1969). Coronary Heart Disease, Stroke, and Aortic Aneurysm. Archives of Environmental Health: An International Journal, 19(2), 167–182.
[clxviii] Hammond, E. C., & Garfinkel, L. (1969). Coronary Heart Disease, Stroke, and Aortic Aneurysm. Archives of Environmental Health: An International Journal, 19(2), 167–182.
[clxix] Aysha Arshad, Anisha Mandava, Ganesh Kamath, Dan Musat, Sudden

Cardiac Death and the Role of Medical Therapy, Progress in Cardiovascular Diseases,

[clxx] Ho CLB, Breslin M, Doust J, et al Effectiveness of blood pressure-lowering drug treatment by levels of absolute risk: post hoc analysis of the Australian National Blood Pressure Study BMJ Open 2018;8:e017723. doi: 10.1136/bmjopen-2017-017723

[clxxi] How Much Is Enough? Efficiency and Medicare Spending in the Last Six Months of Life Author: Jonathan S. Skinner, John Wennberg Chapter URL: http://www.nber.org/chapters/c6763

[clxxii] Mbata G, Chukwuka J. Obstructive sleep apnea hypopnea syndrome. Ann Med Health Sci Res. 2012 Jan;2(1):74-7. doi: 10.4103/2141-9248.96943. PMID: 23209996; PMCID: PMC3507119.

[clxxiii] Karimi M, Hedner J, Häbel H, Nerman O, Grote L. Sleep apnea-related risk of motor vehicle accidents is reduced by continuous positive airway pressure: Swedish Traffic Accident Registry data. Sleep. 2015 Mar 1;38(3):341-9. doi: 10.5665/sleep.4486. PMID: 25325460; PMCID: PMC4335527.

[clxxiv] Tregear S, Reston J, Schoelles K, Phillips B. Obstructive sleep apnea and risk of motor vehicle crash: systematic review and meta-analysis. J Clin Sleep Med. 2009 Dec 15;5(6):573-81. PMID: 20465027; PMCID: PMC2792976.

[clxxv] Benca RM, Obermeyer WH, Thisted RA, Gillin JC. Sleep and psychiatric disorders. A meta-analysis. Arch Gen Psychiatry. 1992;49(8):651–668, discussion 669-670.

[clxxvi] Daches, S., Vine, V., George, C. J., Jennings, J. R., & Kovacs, M. (2020). Sympathetic arousal during the processing of dysphoric affect by youths at high and low familial risk for depression. Psychophysiology.

[clxxvii] Definitions from https://www.mayoclinic.org

[clxxviii] https://www.cdc.gov/diabetes/basics/diabetes.html

[clxxix] Reutrakul, S., & Mokhlesi, B. (2017). Obstructive Sleep Apnea and Diabetes. Chest, 152(5), 1070–1086. doi:10.1016/j.chest.2017.05.00

[clxxx] Bottini P, Redolfi S, Dottorini ML, Tantucci C. Autonomic neuropathy increases the risk of obstructive sleep apnoea in obese diabetes. Respiration. 2008;75:265–71

[clxxxi] Crummy F, Piper AJ, Naughton MT. Obesity and the lung: Obesity and sleep disordered breathing. Thorax. 2008;63:738–46.

[clxxxii] Douglas NJ. Sleep Apnoea. In: Fausi AS, Kasper DL, Longo LD, Braunwald E, Hauser SL, Jameson JL, et al., editors. Harrisons Principles of Internal Medicine. New York: Mc Graw –Hill; 2008. pp. 1665–7.

[clxxxiii] Olson EJ, Moore WR, Morgenthaler TI, Gay PC, Staats BA. Obstructive sleep apnoea hypopnoea syndrome. Mayo Clin Proc. 2003;78:1545–52.

[clxxxiv] Reutrakul, S., & Mokhlesi, B. (2017). Obstructive Sleep Apnea and Diabetes. Chest, 152(5), 1070–1086. doi:10.1016/j.chest.2017.05.0

[clxxxv] Ogden CL, Carroll MD, Lawman HG, et al. Trends in Obesity Prevalence Among Children and Adolescents in the United States, 1988-1994 Through 2013-2014. JAMA. 2016;315(21):2292–2299. doi:10.1001/jama.2016.6361

[clxxxvi] Skinner, A. C., Ravanbakht, S. N., Skelton, J. A., Perrin, E. M., & Armstrong, S. C. (2018). Prevalence of Obesity and Severe Obesity in US Children, 1999–2016. Pediatrics, 141(3), e20173459. doi:10.1542/peds.2017-3459

[clxxxvii] Kim, J., Bhattacharjee, R., Dayyat, E. et al. Increased Cellular Proliferation and Inflammatory Cytokines in Tonsils Derived From Children With Obstructive Sleep Apnea. Pediatr Res 66, 423–428 (2009). https://doi.org/10.1203/PDR.0b013e3181b453e3

[clxxxviii] Amit Kumar Shrivastava, Harsh Vardhan Singh, Arun Raizada, Sanjeev Kumar Singh, C-reactive protein, inflammation and coronary heart disease, The Egyptian Heart Journal, Volume 67, Issue 2, 2015, Pages 89-97,

[clxxxix] Yongjing Zhou, Wei Han, Dandan Gong, Changfeng Man, Yu Fan, Hs-CRP in stroke: A meta-analysis, Clinica Chimica Acta, Volume 453, 2016, Pages 21-27,

[cxc] Dana E. King, Arch G. Mainous, Thomas A. Buchanan, William S. Pearson; C-Reactive Protein and Glycemic Control in Adults With Diabetes . Diabetes Care 1 May 2003; 26 (5): 1535–1539

[cxci] Li, J., Zhao, F., Wang, Y. et al. Gut microbiota dysbiosis contributes to the development of hypertension. Microbiome 5, 14 (2017)

[cxcii] Bartolomaeus H, Balogh A, Yakoub M, Homann S, Markó L, Höges S, Tsvetkov D, Krannich A, Wundersitz S, Avery EG, Haase N, Kräker K, Hering L, Maase M, Kusche-Vihrog K, Grandoch M, Fielitz J, Kempa S, Gollasch M, Zhumadilov Z, Kozhakhmetov S, Kushugulova A, Eckardt KU, Dechend R, Rump LC, Forslund SK, Müller DN, Stegbauer J, Wilck N. Short-Chain Fatty Acid Propionate Protects From Hypertensive Cardiovascular Damage. Circulation. 2019 Mar 12;139(11):1407-1421. doi: 10.1161/CIRCULATIONAHA.118.036652. PMID: 30586752; PMCID: PMC6416008.

[cxciii] Martinez Jason E., Kahana Doron D., Ghuman Simran, Wilson Haley P., Wilson Julian, Kim Samuel C. J., Lagishetty Venu, Jacobs Jonathan P., Sinha-Hikim Amiya P., Friedman Theodore C. Unhealthy Lifestyle and Gut Dysbiosis: A Better Understanding of the Effects of Poor Diet and Nicotine on the Intestinal Microbiome Frontiers in Endocrinology Vol 12 2021

[cxciv] Ko CY, Liu QQ, Su HZ, Zhang HP, Fan JM, Yang JH, Hu AK, Liu YQ, Chou D, Zeng YM. Gut microbiota in obstructive sleep apnea-hypopnea syndrome: disease-related dysbiosis and metabolic comorbidities. Clin Sci (Lond). 2019 Apr 12;133(7):905-917. doi: 10.1042/CS20180891. PMID: 30957778; PMCID: PMC6465302.

[cxcv] Ko CY, Fan JM, Hu AK, Su HZ, Yang JH, Huang LM, Yan FR, Zhang

HP, Zeng YM. Disruption of sleep architecture in Prevotella enterotype of patients with obstructive sleep apnea-hypopnea syndrome. Brain Behav. 2019 May;9(5):e01287. doi: 10.1002/brb3.1287. Epub 2019 Apr 8. PMID: 30957979; PMCID: PMC6520469.

[cxcvi] Zeng X, Guo R, Dong M, Zheng J, Lin H, Lu H. Contribution of TLR4 signaling in intermittent hypoxia-mediated atherosclerosis progression. J Transl Med. 2018 Apr 19;16(1):106. doi: 10.1186/s12967-018-1479-6. PMID: 29673358; PMCID: PMC5907703.

[cxcvii] Kyle Hoffman, MD, Emad Mansoor, MD, Muhammad Siyab Panhwar, MD, Miguel Regueiro, MD, Gregory Cooper, MD, Taha Qazi, MD, Prevalence of Obstructive Sleep Apnea Is Increased in Patients With Inflammatory Bowel Disease: A Large, Multi-Network Study, Crohn's & Colitis 360, Volume 4, Issue 3, July 2022,

[cxcviii] Zeng X, Guo R, Dong M, Zheng J, Lin H, Lu H. Contribution of TLR4 signaling in intermittent hypoxia-mediated atherosclerosis progression. J Transl Med. 2018 Apr 19;16(1):106. doi: 10.1186/s12967-018-1479-6. PMID: 29673358; PMCID: PMC5907703.

[cxcix] Schellekens DH, Grootjans J, Dello SA, van Bijnen AA, van Dam RM, Dejong CH, Derikx JP, Buurman WA. Plasma intestinal fatty acid-binding protein levels correlate with morphologic epithelial intestinal damage in a human translational ischemia-reperfusion model. J Clin Gastroenterol. 2014 Mar;48(3):253-60. doi: 10.1097/MCG.0b013e3182a87e3e. PMID: 24100750.

[cc] Lee DW, Kim JG, Yang YM. Influence of mouth breathing on atopic dermatitis risk and oral health in children: A population-based cross-sectional study. J Dent Sci. 2021 Jan;16(1):178-185. doi: 10.1016/j.jds.2020.06.014. Epub 2020 Jun 22. PMID: 33384795; PMCID: PMC7770290.

[cci] Katz, E. S., Mitchell, R. B., & D'Ambrosio, C. M. (2012). Obstructive Sleep Apnea in Infants. American Journal of Respiratory and Critical Care Medicine, 185(8), 805–816. doi:10.1164/rccm.201108-1455ci

[ccii] Rhoads, J. M., Collins, J., Fatheree, N. Y., Hashmi, S. S., Taylor, C. M., Luo, M., ... Liu, Y. (2018). Infant Colic Represents Gut Inflammation and Dysbiosis. The Journal of Pediatrics.

[i] Prevalence estimates range from rare to 17% of the general population Hacmisch B, et. al. Immunal acaa37a97-aos Malderings Gil. et al. PLoS One aug.S(y) a76a,

[ii] Theoharides TC. Neuroendocrinology of mast cells: Challenges and controversies. Exp Dermatol. 2017 Sep;26(9):751-759. doi: 10.1111/exd.13288. Epub 2017 Apr 2. PMID: 28094875.

[iii] Theoharis C. Theoharides, Souad Enakuaa, Nikolaos Sismanopoulos, Shahrzad Asadi, Evangelos C. Papadimas, Asimenia Angelidou, Konstantinos-Dionysios Alysandratos, Contribution of stress to asthma worsening through

mast cell activation, Annals of Allergy, Asthma & Immunology, Volume 109, Issue 1, 2012, Pages 14-19,

[iv] Afrin LB, Self S, Menk J, Lazarchick J. Characterization of Mast Cell Activation Syndrome. Am J Med Sci. 2017 Mar;353(3):207-215. doi: 10.1016/j.amjms.2016.12.013. Epub 2016 Dec 16. PMID: 28262205; PMCID: PMC5341697.

[v] https://www.jacionline.org/action/showPdf?pii=S0091-6749%2816%2932061-9 Inflammatory mediators released from mast cells recruited into the tonsil induce the development of obstructive sleep apnea Jai Youl Ro1,et al Journey Of Allergy and Clinical immunology.

[vi] Mast Cell Survival and Mediator Secretion in Response to Hypoxia Magdalena Gulliksson, Ricardo F. S. Carvalho, Erik Ulleras, Gunnar Nilsson August 23, 2010 PLOS one

[vii] The Journal of Clinical Investigation Mast cell hyperactivity underpins the development of oxygen-induced retinopathy Volume 127 Number 11 November 2017 Kenshiro Matsuda,1 Noriko Okamoto,2 Masatoshi Kondo,3 Peter D. Arkwright,4 Kaoru Karasawa,1 Saori Ishizaka,1 Shinichi Yokota,2 Akira Matsuda,2 Kyungsook Jung,1 Kumiko Oida,1 Yosuke Amagai,1,5 Hyosun Jang,1 Eiichiro Noda,6 Ryota Kakinuma,7 Koujirou Yasui,7 Uiko Kaku,7 Yasuo Mori,8 Nobuyuki Onai,9 Toshiaki Ohteki,9 Akane Tanaka,1,7 and Hiroshi Matsuda1,2

[viii] The Last Surgeon Lweis Newberg MD (15 October 2008) ISBN-10 : 1436365082 ISBN-13 : 978-1436365086

[ix] Öztürk L, Ünal M, Tamer L, Çelikoğlu F. The Association of the Severity of Obstructive Sleep Apnea With Plasma Leptin Levels. Arch Otolaryngol Head Neck Surg. 2003;129(5):538–540. doi:10.1001/archotol.129.5.538

[x] Leptin Prevents Respiratory Depression in Obesity CHRISTOPHER P. O'DONNELL, CHARLES D. SCHAUB, ABBY S. HAINES, DAN E. BERKOWITZ, CLARKE G. TANKERSLEY, ALAN R. SCHWARTZ, and PHILIP L. SMITH American Journal of Respiratory and Critical Care Medicine May 1999, pages 1365- 1659

[xi] REVIEW article Front. Immunol., 06 October 2020 Sec. Cytokines and Soluble Mediators in Immunity Volume 11 - 2020 | https://doi.org/10.3389/fimmu.2020.580378 Neuropeptide Y Is an Immunomodulatory Factor: Direct and Indirect Wei-can Chen1, Yi-bin Liu1, Wei-feng Liu1, Ying-ying Zhou1, He-fan He1* and Shu Lin

[xii] Conti P, Pregliasco FE, Bellomo RG, Gallenga CE, Caraffa A, Kritas SK, Lauritano D, Ronconi G. Mast Cell Cytokines IL-1, IL-33, and IL-36 Mediate Skin Inflammation in Psoriasis: A Novel Therapeutic Approach with the Anti-Inflammatory Cytokines IL-37, IL-38, and IL-1Ra. Int J Mol Sci. 2021 Jul 28;22(15):8076. doi: 10.3390/ijms22158076. PMID: 34360845; PMCID: PMC8348737.

[xiii] Moldofsky H, Lue FA, Davidson JR, Gorczynski R. Effects of sleep deprivation on human immune functions. FASEB J. 1989 Jun;3(8):1972-7. doi: 10.1096/fasebj.3.8.2785942. PMID: 2785942.

[xiv] Sleep, 20(11):1027-103, American Sleep Disorders Association and Sleep Research Society . Ruth M, Benca and tJose Quintans Sleep and Host Defences: A Review

Acknowledgments

This book would not have been possible without the love support and encouragement of my wife Nicky and the trials and tribulations of my children. They taught me to never give up, there is always an answer, just keep looking.

I would like to also pay tribute to the essential work of Emeritus Professor Louise Nicholson, Comp of the NZ Order of Merit. Her research changed my life and created the lens that I view all health issues through. Small changes and alterations can have far reaching unexpected consequences. Just because the effect is not obvious, does not mean it's not there.

I am made better for the Education of Professor Mel Sydney-Smith and Professor Theodore Carrick. Both have dedicated there lives to improving human health and pushing the boundaries of understanding.

Finally, I'd like to thank Stephanie Willis for introducing me to Functional Neurology and Samantha Haitsma and for triggering the thought to undertake this journey.

Thank you to all the other unnamed people who helped me the bring this information into being.

Milton Keynes UK
Ingram Content Group UK Ltd.
UKHW022054120624
444052UK00013B/627

9 780645 830408